The
Psychiatric
Interview

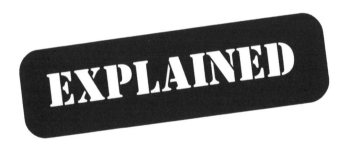

EXPLAINED

David J. Robinson, M.D., F.R.C.P.C.
Diplomate of the American Board of
Psychiatry & Neurology

Rapid Psychler Press

Suite 374
3560 Pine Grove Ave.
Port Huron, Michigan
USA 48060

Suite 203
1673 Richmond St.
London, Ontario
Canada N6G 2N3

Toll Free Phone   888-PSY-CHLE (888-779-2453)
Toll Free Fax   888-PSY-CHLR (888-779-2457)
Outside the U.S. & Canada — Fax 519-675-0610
website www.psychler.com
email   rapid@psychler.com

ISBN 1-894328-21-3
Printed in the United States of America
© 2000, Rapid Psychler Press
First Edition, First Printing

Dedication

This book is dedicated to my sister
Dr. Donna L. Robinson

Acknowledgments

I am indebted to the following individuals for their unfailing support in assisting me with this text.

- **Brian & Fanny Chapman**
- **Monty & Lil Robinson**
- **Lisa & Cathy Burgard**
- **Nicole & Mark Kennedy**
- **Dr. Donna Robinson & Dr. Robert Bauer**
- **Dean Avola**
- **Brad Groshok**

I would also like to thank the following people for their helpful reviews of this manuscript.

- **Lisa & Cathy Burgard**
- **Tom Norry, B.Sc.N.**
- **Thomas Gantert, B.Sc.N.**
- **Dr. Sandra Northcott**
- **Dr. Lisa Bogue**
- **Dr. Michelle Kelly**

Rapid Psychler Press

produces books and presentation media that are:

• comprehensively researched
• well organized
• formatted for ease of use
• reasonably priced
• clinically oriented, and
• include humor that enhances education, and that neither demeans patients nor the efforts of those who treat them

Table of Contents

Publication Notes

Terminology
Throughout this book, the term "patient" refers to people who are suffering and seek help. The term further describes those who bear pain without complaint or anger. The terms "consumer" or "consumer-survivor" reflect an unfortunate trend that is pejorative towards mental health care, labeling it as if it were a trade or business instead of a profession. These terms are also ambiguous, as it is not clear what is being "consumed" or "survived."

Graphics
All of the illustrations in this book are original works of art commissioned by Rapid Psychler Press and are a signature feature of our publications. Rapid Psychler Press makes available an entire library of color illustrations (including those from this book) as 35mm slides and overhead transparencies. These images are available for viewing and can be purchased from our website — **www.psychler.com**

The images from our color library may be used for presentations. We request that you respect our copyright and do not reproduce these images in any form for any purpose at any time.

Bolded Terms
Throughout this book, various terms appear in bolded text which allows for ease of identification. Most of these terms are defined in this text. Some, however, are only mentioned because a detailed description is beyond the scope of this book. Fuller explanations of all of the bolded terms can be found in standard reference texts.

1/ *The Psychiatric Interview*

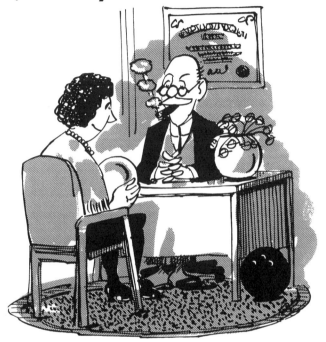

Introduction

Clinical interviewing is the single most important skill required in psychiatry. The interview is the principal means for gaining an understanding of a patient's difficulties. This understanding leads to a diagnostic formulation and subsequent treatment plan. The assessment process in psychiatry relies primarily on the interviewing and observational skills of practitioners because there is no lab test, tissue diagnosis or imaging method available to confirm a psychiatric diagnosis.

The interview can be defined as "the skill of encouraging disclosure of personal information for a specific professional purpose" (McCready, 1986), and serves a variety of functions:

- Collecting clinical information in an efficient manner
- Eliciting emotions, feelings, and attitudes
- Establishing a doctor-patient relationship and developing rapport
- Generating and testing a set of hypotheses to arrive at a **preferred diagnosis**, accompanied by a list of other conditions (called a **differential diagnosis**) which must be considered
- Determining areas for further investigation
- Developing a treatment plan

Interviewing is not simply the task of taking a history. Rather, it is the process of determining which illness the patient has, and understanding how he or she has been affected by it. Far more than a series of questions, a well-conducted interview yields information that helps develop an individualized approach for treating the patient.

A careful history contributes more to determining a diagnosis in medically ill patients than does the physical examination which, in turn, is of greater usefulness than laboratory testing (Anfinson, 1992; Hampton, 1975).

Anatomy of the Psychiatric Interview

In 1996, the APA published a set of practice guidelines for general psychiatric evaluation of adults. The following "domains of evaluation" comprise a complete psychiatric interview:

A. Reason for the Evaluation
B. History of the Present Illness
C. Past Psychiatric History
D. General Medical History

E. History of Substance Use
F. Psychosocial/Developmental History (Personal History)
G. Social History
H. Occupational History
 I. Family History
J. Review of Symptoms
K. Physical Examination
L. Mental Status Examination (MSE)
      Appearance
      Behavior
      Cooperation
      Speech
      Thought (Content & Process)
      Affect
      Mood
      Perception
      Level of Consciousness
      Insight & Judgment
      Cognitive Functioning & Sensorium
      Knowledge Base
      Endings — Suicidal & Homicidal Ideation
      Reliability of Information
M. Functional Assessment
N. Diagnostic Tests
O. Information Derived From The Interview Process

Functions of the Interview

Nurcombe (1982) indicated that interviewers must develop an understanding (sometimes called a **formulation**) of two domains, **nosologic** and **dynamic**. Nosological refers to the exercise of figuring out which condition(s) the patient suffers from. The dynamic domain involves an application of eliciting the biopsychosocial aspects of the patient's illness:

- In what way(s) was the patient **predisposed** to getting this condition?
- What **precipitating** factors caused this illness to emerge at this time?

- What factors **perpetuate** this illness in its current form?
- What **protective factors** (strengths, supports, resources, etc.) does this patient have?

Often, these parameters are divided into biological, social, and psychological components. A grid can be constructed to aid the process of dynamic formulation:

	Biological	Social	Psychological
Predisposing			
Precipitating			
Perpetuating			
Protective			

While the **nosologic** or **diagnostic formulation** can be completed relatively early in the interview, the **dynamic formulation** can take an extended period of time. The interview can be considered to have two tasks: making a diagnosis, and understanding the patient's psychosocial milieu. The sections of the interview particularly relevant to these areas are as follows:

Diagnostic Formulation
Reason for Referral
History of Present Illness
Psychiatric History
General Medical History
History of Substance Use
Review of Symptoms
Mental Status Exam

Dynamic Formulation
Identifying Factors
Personal History
Family History
Social History
Occupational History

What Are the Consequences of Poor Interviewing Skills?

The benefits of a well-conducted, thorough, and empathic interview are intuitively obvious. The effects of poorly conducted interviews are extensive and unfortunate:

- Patient dissatisfaction (Reynolds, 1978)
- Poor compliance (Ley, 1982)
- Missed diagnoses (Goldberg, 1980)
- Inappropriate treatment (McCready, 1986)
- Formal complaints (Fletcher, 1980)
- Increased litigation (Carroll, 1979)

Poor interviewing skills also impact on students and residents. During training, students and residents are much more likely to fail rotations and examinations (such as the American Board of Psychiatry & Neurology Part II Exam) as a result of deficient interviewing skills. Students failing psychiatric examinations in medical school may develop a bias against the specialty, which can even extend to patients with mental illnesses encountered on medical or surgical wards. Residents failing rotations or examinations may need to defer their career plans, and some change programs after encountering such difficulties.

Clinical Problem Solving/ Hypothesis Generation

- Evaluate salient cues (hospital record, reason for referral to psychiatry, medical records (old chart), initial observations of the patient, etc.) to develop clinical inferences from this preliminary information
- Designate data as a sign or symptom of an illness (i.e. does the sign or symptom fall out of the range of typical or common experiences, and if so, does this qualify as a diagnostic criterion?
- Combine inferences and clinical information to group the pertinent manifestations into a preliminary array of **diag-**

nostic hypotheses (a list of possible conditions); this can be based on as little as one sign or symptom

- Investigate hypotheses by requesting more information (note that discrepancies, inconsistencies, gaps, and contrasts also provide useful information); weigh the positive and negative evidence
- Recognize and evaluate the material from the interview; revise the diagnostic impression based on new information (e.g. strengthen a current diagnosis, weaken/ discard a diagnosis, add a new diagnosis to the hypothesis)
- Use the revised hypothetical array to guide the search for more information (this also includes a review of systems where screening questions (probes) are used to check for associated or rare conditions)
- Use probability estimation to arrive at a **preferred diagnosis** (this would have the maximum number of positive features, and the greatest difference between positive and negative evidence), and a list of other conditions (**differential diagnosis**) in descending order of likelihood
- Complete the interview to understand the relevant psychosocial factors
- Develop a comprehensive management plan based on the diagnosis and biopsychosocial factors elucidated in the interview

Hypotheses are generated early in the interview with limited data available. In a group of psychiatrists studied by Gauron (1966), the most efficient diagnosticians generated hypotheses after two pieces of information were given (e.g. age and reason for referral), and needed only 8 to 14 bits total to arrive at a diagnosis (the least efficient interviewers needed up to 36). Maguire (1976) observed a group of senior medical students conducting a standardized 15-minute interview. In this time period, students elicited an average of 14 useful pieces of information, which was estimated to be about one-third of the data available under the imposed time constraints.

In other studies, it was found that physicians generated their initial hypotheses in less than one minute, containing an average of six possible diagnoses (Feightner, 1975 & Barrows, 1979). At just five minutes into the interview, they had finalized their hypotheses about which illnesses they thought the patient might have. Over half the relevant information was obtained in the first quarter of the interview. By necessity, formulation must begin early. In many situations, interviewers do not have the chance to spend extended periods of time with patients. In situations where a specific task is required (i.e. emergency room interviews triaging patients; consultation interviews focusing on the question posed by the consultee), hypothesis generation begins immediately upon speaking with patients.

Structured Interviews

Signs and symptoms in psychiatry ultimately are subjective determinations which is probably the single most perplexing aspect for students. Concepts, definitions, and diagnostic practices vary between psychiatrists. One of the driving forces behind the formation of the first edition of the **Diagnostic and Statistical Manual of Mental Disorders (DSM)** in 1952 was the need for standardization. For example, historically the term "schizophrenia" was applied to a diverse number of conditions, making research efforts and communication between psychiatrists very difficult. It was not until the DSM-III was published in 1980 that individual criteria for psychiatric disorders were identified. The **World Health Organization (WHO)** publishes a similar set of diagnostic criteria called the **International Classification of Diseases**, currently in its tenth edition (**ICD-10**). Greater integration between the DSM and the ICD classification systems is planned.

With the advent of a standardized set of diagnostic criteria, attention began to focus on valid and reliable ways of collecting data — structured interviews. There has been widespread appreciation of, and acceptance for, the development of structured interviews extending back over decades (Rose, 1968; Kramer, 1969; Zubin, 1969). A standardized assessment tool would go a long way to diminishing the variation in methodology, training, and emphasis seen in clinical psychiatry.

A distinction needs to be drawn between a structured interview and a questionnaire. Structured interviews are generally composed of closed-ended questions (ones prompting patients for a discrete answer, such as yes or no), but interviewers are able to ask supplemental questions until a satisfactory understanding has been reached.

A number of structured interviews are currently available (see below). They vary in scope (e.g. the number of conditions they are designed to diagnose) and content (which criteria are used to pose the questions: DSM, ICD, Research Diagnostic Criteria, etc.). Examples are:

- Structured Clinical Interview for DSM-IV Axis I Disorders (SCID-I)
- Structured Clinical Interview for DSM-IV Axis II Personality Disorders (SCID-II)
- Structured Clinical Interview for DSM-IV Dissociative Disorders (SCID-D)

One of the concerns about the widespread use of structured interviews is that the focus centers on eliciting diagnostic findings at the expense of the psychosocial and emotional factors. Saghir (1971) compared a structured interview to the typical, or free-style interview, and found the former to be more comprehensive in detecting and documenting psychiatric illness. He noted that interviewers using the standardized instrument displayed less of an interest in the emotional state of the patient, and more of an interest in completing the assessment. The main advantage to the free-style approach was that it allowed interviewers to change their focus from diagnosis to therapy if the situation warranted such a shift.

References

American Psychiatric Association
Diagnostic and Statistical Manual of Mental Disorders, 1952
Diagnostic and Statistical Manual of Mental Disorders, 3rd Edition, 1980
Diagnostic and Statistical Manual of Mental Disorders, 4th Edition, 1994
Practice Guidelines: Psychiatric Evaluation of Adults, 1996
American Psychiatric Association, Washington D.C.

T.J. Anfinson & R.G. Kathol
Screening Laboratory Evaluation in Psychiatric Patients: A Review
General Hospital Psychiatry 14: p. 248 — 257, 1992

H.S. Barrows
An Overview of Medical Problem Solving
University of Vermont Office of Continuing Medical Education, Burlington, Vermont, 1979

J.G. Carroll & J. Monroe
Teaching Medical Interviewing
Journal of Medical Education 54: p. 498, 1979

J.W. Feightner, G.R. Norman, H.S. Barrows & V.R. Neufeld
A Comparison of the Clinical Methods of Primary Care Physicians
Association of American Medical Colleges, Washington D.C., 1975

C. Fletcher
Listening and Talking to Patients III. The Exposition
British Medical Journal 281: p. 994 — 996, 1980

E.F. Gauron & J.K. Dickinson
Diagnostic Decision-Making in Psychiatry I: Information Usage & II: Diagnostic Styles
Archives of General Psychiatry 14: p. 225 — 232 & p. 233 — 237, 1966

D.P. Goldberg, J.J. Steel, C. Smith & L. Sprireg
Training Family Doctors to Recognize Psychiatric Illness
Lancet ii: p. 521 — 523, 1980

G.R. Hampton, M.T.G. Harrison, J.R.A. Mitchell, J.S. Pritchard & C. Seymour
Relative Contributions of History Taking, Physical Examination and Laboratory Investigations to Diagnosis and Management of Medical Patients
British Medical Journal 2: p. 486 — 7, 1975

M. Kramer
Application of Mental Health Statistics
World Health Organization, Geneva, 1969

P. Ley
Satisfaction, Compliance and Communications
British Journal of Clinical Psychology 21: p. 241 — 254, 1982

G.P. Maguire & D.R. Rutter
History Taking For Medical Students: Evaluation of a Training Program
Lancet ii: p. 558 — 560, 1976

J.R. McCready & F M. Waring
Interviewing Skills in Relation to Psychiatric Residency
Canadian Journal of Psychiatry 31: p. 317 — 322, 1986

B. Nurcombe & I. Fitzhenry-Coor
How Do Psychiatrists Think? Clinical Reasoning in the Psychiatric Interview
Australian & New Zealand Journal of Psychiatry 16: p. 13 — 24, 1982

M. Reynolds
No News is Bad News: Patients' Views About Communication in Hospital
British Medical Journal 1: p. 1673 — 1676, 1978

G.A. Rose & H. Blackburn
Cardiovascular Surgery Methods, Monograph Series 56
World Health Organization, Geneva, 1968

M. Saghir
A Comparison of Some Aspects of Structured and Unstructured Psychiatric Interviews
American Journal of Psychiatry 128: p. 180 — 184, 1971

J. Zubin
Cross-National Study of Diagnosis of the Mental Disorders: Methodology and Planning
American Journal of Psychiatry 125 (April Supplement): p. 12 — 20, 1969

2/ *The Interview Process*

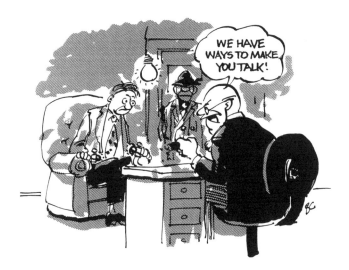

Introduction

Content refers to *what* information is obtained in an interview, while **process** refers to *how* the information is obtained. Process can also be thought of as style or technique. It is as important to successful interviewing as is content, otherwise assessments would be reduced to completing questionnaires.

It is entirely possible to conduct an interview that is adequate in terms of content, but misses the mark in terms of establishing a relationship with the patient. This can have disastrous consequences, such as poor patient compliance and cancellation of follow-up visits. A leading cause of failed examinations in psychiatry is that students have a rigid, mechanical interview style that focuses primarily on phenomenology.

The psychiatric interview was designed to obtain and organize information essential to the task of treating mental illness. As such, the interview is an artificial construct, of which patients know little to nothing. Because we ask for highly personal and sensitive information in a manner of our design, it behooves us to facilitate this information exchange with the utmost respect and caring for our patients. A well-conducted interview has the following features:

- The air of a polite, objective inquiry is maintained (e.g. using Ms., Mr., Mrs. to address patients)
- Interviewers demonstrate curiosity and acceptance
- Patients understand the purpose, duration, etc.
- Patients' comfort is considered
- Patients have the chance to speak about what concerns them
- There are no outside intrusions or distractions
- Changes in topic are effected smoothly
- Lengthy periods of silence are avoided
- The flow and rhythm characteristic of a conversation develops
- Information about both facts and feelings is obtained

Gaining facility with interviewing processes takes years to develop. The reader is referred to three texts that are of particular assistance: Shea (1998), Othmer & Othmer (1994), and Morrison (1995). Two aspects of process are presented in this chapter:

- Empathy, rapport & therapeutic alliance
- Types of interview questions and interventions

Empathy, Rapport & Therapeutic Alliance

One definition of **empathy** is "making a connection to the emotional state of another person." A second is "a form of cognition that enables one to comprehend another person's subjective experiences from his or her own perspective"

(Campbell, 1996). Empathy is akin to the saying "walk a mile in my shoes" in that you put yourself in a patient's place to try and comprehend the situation. Empathy is different than sympathy, which is often expressed as pity. The distinction may be a subtle one, as sympathy does have a place in the interview process. However, Rutter (1981) reported that a certain level of sympathy was desirable, while excessive amounts work against the interviewer in terms of eliciting feelings. Morrison (1995) suggests that interviewers can maintain an empathic focus by keeping the following thought in mind: *What would it be like to be this patient talking with me now?* Empathy can perhaps be most clearly demonstrated by the way we act towards a friend going through a difficult period. We would listen, show concern, offer support, and try to find a way to help. While we have boundaries as professionals, our natural and humanistic responses help us find empathic ways to connect with patients.

A common misapplication of empathy is the farcical "I feel your pain" which appears in the popular media. Shea (1998) reminds us that patients are looking for someone who can understand their feelings, not feel as they do. It is important to maintain a personal perspective in expressing empathy, as objectivity is one of the hallmarks of a mental health professional.

A literal definition of **rapport** is "a bringing back," which refers to harmonious relationships with patients. Rapport builds by treating patients respectfully, being interested in their problems, and demonstrating competence in your craft. This perpetual curiosity has been referred to as an **analytic attitude**, signifying an interest in all elements of the person, with a continual refinement in understanding his or her difficulties. Gabbard (1982) illustrated the need for continual attention to the interview process by examining the last statements patients made as they left psychotherapy sessions. These statements have been called **exit lines** or **doorknob comments**, and may reveal more about what is going on in the patient's mind than the content of the entire session. For example, a patient who tells a joke on the way out of the room may be compensating for being "boring" and has to leave the clinician with some reason to want to book another appointment.

Developing rapport is essential to developing a **therapeutic alliance**, which is an understanding that you are working with the patient for the reduction of symptoms and the enhancement of quality of life. The patient has accepted you as an ally in the battle against the illness. It is the strength of the therapeutic alliance that brings patients back for appointments, gives them the willingness to try a new medication, helps them weather a difficult psychotherapy session, etc.

Calm and friendly acknowledgment of a painful or frightening emotional state in itself has therapeutic effects, and helps patients feel understood and accepted. Empathy can be demonstrated in many ways, including the following:

Explaining the Interview Process
- State your name, your position in the department, the role others in the room have (e.g. observer, supervisor, etc.), and the anticipated (or available) time for the assessment
- Ask the patient what his or her expectations are for the interview
- Outline the purpose of the interview and the areas of information you'll be requesting (e.g. personal history, family history, etc.)
- Indicate if you will be seeing the patient again (e.g. to continue in psychotherapy) or if this is a one-time interview (e.g. a consultation request from a family doctor)
- Ask if the patient needs a drink, a washroom break, an ashtray (if smoking is allowed), etc.

- Check to see that the patient is comfortable with the arrangement you have outlined and ask if it is OK to proceed (you may also need to inquire about informed consent, particularly if the interview is recorded)

Easing Into the Interview
- Ask a few general questions to "warm up" the interaction; this can center on identifying factors such as full name, age, and occupation; queries about difficulties finding the hospital; or if possible, establishing some common or neutral ground
- Let patients have free rein to speak about what is on their minds at the beginning of the interview

Facilitating the Flow of Information
- Establish and maintain good eye contact
- Nod your head; show an expression of interest
- Make interjections such as or "Uh-huh" or "Go ahead"
- Lean forward in your chair (this indicates interest)
- Take as few notes as possible
- Exude a calm, neutral acceptance of what patients tell you

Connecting with the Patient's Emotions
- Recognize and immediately respond to expressions of emotion
- Notice nonverbal cues (e.g. facial expression, posture)
- Make direct requests for patients to express their feelings (assess their suffering)

Demonstrating Your Expertise
- Intermittently clarify your understanding of the patient's difficulties
- Establish and maintain control of the interview — patients often feel as if things around them are chaotic and respond well to structure

- Convey that you are familiar with problems like the ones you are being told about
- Demonstrate your knowledge of the condition and related features by taking a full history — patients are impressed by thoroughness
- Instill a sense of perspective on the illness and hope for the future (in that efforts will be made to help the person, and that most patients have at least some response to treatment)

More About Empathy

While some students have a natural capacity for empathy, many can learn to be more empathic. In order for empathy to be effective, it must be genuine, spontaneous, and accurate. There are some people who have difficulty exuding warmth in interview situations. Othmer & Othmer (1994) indicate that focused attention and appropriate questions convey interest, and are preferable to phony-sounding or rehearsed attempts at empathy. Being empathic does not mean that other aspects of the interview can be overlooked. Professional boundaries, time limits, and structure are all crucial to successful interviewing.

Types of Interview Questions

The art of questioning takes many years to refine. Cox, Rutter & Holbrook (1981) reported that in order to obtain good quality data, students asked almost twice as many questions as did experienced interviewers. In addition to the number of questions asked, the timing and wording of questions improves with experience. "High yield" questions are important because they give patients more time to talk. The most common types of interview questions are as follows:

A/ Open-Ended Questions
These are questions that give direction as to the topic you're

interested in with an "open end" to the amount of information requested.

Example: *What difficulties caused you to come to the hospital today?*

Advantages: Open-ended questions give patients the chance to tell you what is most important to them which is usually a spontaneous report about their problems. In this way, open-ended questions act as a projective test in that they reveal what is on patients' minds. These types of questions facilitate the flow of detailed information. Open-ended questions aid in the development of rapport because patients are allowed to express themselves in an uninterrupted manner. While patients are answering these types of questions, you have the opportunity to begin **hypothesis generation** and complete a significant portion of the **mental status examination (MSE)**.

Disadvantages: Open-ended questions can elicit replies that are lengthy and provide scant information for the purposes of the interview. Patients can head off onto new topics that are unrelated to their reason for seeking help (**tangentiality**), or eventually address your question after considerable intervening information has been given (**circumstantiality**). Interrupting patients in the middle of answering open-ended questions poses a problem for some interviewers.

B/ Multiple Choice Questions
These questions begin to introduce some structure to the patient's responses by indicating the range or type of information you are seeking.

Example: *Do you have trouble falling asleep, staying asleep, waking up too early, or with some other aspect of your sleep?*

Advantage: These questions can be asked in a way that gives

patients the chance to direct the interview (e.g. the last option from the above question). By setting a range of responses, the patient is guided to provide information which is on topic.

Disadvantage: Patients may find it confusing to keep all the options in mind. There may also be a selection bias in choosing either the first or last item (primacy and recency of memory). The patient may also wish to say something that falls outside the parameters you've set, but feels reluctant to mention it because it wasn't an option.

C/ Directive or Focused Questions
These questions ask for specific information, but encourage a more detailed reply than a closed-ended question.

Example: *How does your mood vary throughout the day?*

Advantages: These questions narrow the focus more than open-ended questions. They are often used as follow-up questions after open-ended ones. Focused questions get more information about areas that you have indicated are important.

Disadvantages: Some patients may feel they have not had enough of a chance to say what was on their minds.

D/ Closed-Ended Questions
These are questions that ask for specific information, often requiring only a single word answer (e.g. yes or no).

Example: *Have you ever been admitted to hospital for psychiatric reasons?*

Advantages: Closed-ended questions elicit brief answers that are on topic. Because the interviewer sets the parameters of the closed-ended question, they are used to address points that patients omit in answers to more open-ended questions. Considerable progress can be made quickly in selected areas with closed-ended questions.

Disadvantages: Closed-ended questions lead patients and inhibit the spontaneous flow of information. Some patients may not be able to, or not wish to, give such a brief answer to a question. Closed-ended questions can seem like an interrogation if too many are asked in a row. Also, the manner in which questions are posed can lead the patient into giving a false answer. Because of the quick response, interviewers must be ready with the next question, leaving little time to process what the patient just said.

E/ Double Questions
Double questions are those that pose two options simultaneously.

Example of a poorly composed double question: *Do you ever have visions or believe things that other people disagree with?*

Example of a more thoughtfully composed double question: *Do you ever have visions, or see things that other people can't see?*

Advantages: Double questions resemble directive/ focused questions if the two options are closely related. Such questions can help cover ground more quickly.

Disadvantages: The answer to a poorly composed double question is either ambiguous (e.g. an answer of yes or no doesn't clarify which option is being addressed), or the patient has to answer each aspect separately, which takes effort. If the patient does not take the time to clarify an answer, the data obtained from the interview is less reliable.

F/ Leading Questions

These questions "lead" patients towards an answer that you already have in mind. Leading questions are used frequently by lawyers during cross-examination in order to direct testimony to a particular conclusion (which of course helps the lawyer's argument).

Example: *You've never used street drugs, have you?*

Advantages: Leading questions are not a good way of obtaining unbiased information, but the two main uses of this technique are as follows:

First, leading questions are useful in summing up information already obtained in the interview. For example:

Interviewer: *Let's see, you've told me that you've felt depressed for one month, but in that time you haven't been on any spending sprees or had bursts of energy —*
Patient: *No.*
Interviewer: *. . . or been using any street drugs —*
Patient: *No.*
Interviewer: *. . . or been suffering from any medical illnesses?*
Patient: *No.*

Secondly, leading questions can be of use in guiding patients towards a conclusion, particularly one that is in their best interests. This technique, called **Socratic dialogue**, is used in **cognitive therapy**.

Questions are not used to trap or attack patients, but to assess the consequences of maintaining their maladaptive thoughts or behaviors. Accordingly, questions must be posed sensitively so patients can look at the issue as objectively and non-defensively as possible. For example:

Dr. Eager: *Mr. Crammer, we've talked previously about your request for prescription medication to help you through exams —*
Mr. Crammer: *Yes.*
Dr. Eager: *. . . and you understand that these medications do not have a predictable action on memory, and can backfire and actually impair your performance.*
Mr. Crammer: *I guess so.*
Dr. Eager: *Under these circumstances, is it not to your advantage to write your exams with a clear head and not take the chance of having a bad reaction to medications?*
Mr. Crammer: *I suppose you're right. I'll go home and start preparing for tomorrow's final exam.*

Disadvantages: Asking questions in a manner that suggests a particular response does not assist the process of uncovering accurate information. Leading questions should largely be avoided, but do at times serve a purpose (see also the Substance Use Chapter).

Types of Interventions
In addition to asking questions, there are several other interventions that facilitate the flow of the interview. Patients vary widely in the cues they give concerning their inner feelings, so the interviewer must be capable of using a range of techniques to elicit emotions. Many of these techniques are used in psychotherapy. The only significant disadvantage to these interventions is that they may be used at an inopportune time during the interview.

G/ Clarification
The interviewer asks for more information from the patient to clarify his or her responses. In many situations, patients are distracted, upset, or not thinking clearly, and this is reflected in their answers. In particular, concentration and memory prob-

lems accompany many mental illnesses, and are diminished when people are distracted by being in the midst of a psycho-social crisis.

Example: *I know you've told me a lot about your relationship with your husband, but I need to ask you exactly when you felt he was becoming distant towards you.*

H/ Confrontation
In confronting patients, you draw their attention to a particular behavior that is obstructing the interview (**resistance**). Patients may or may not be aware of the behavior you are pointing out. **Ego defenses** are unconscious mechanisms that protect against emotionally painful situations, such as blaming someone else for one's own forbidden wishes (**projection**) or transferring one's anger into socially acceptable outlets like contact sports (**sublimation**). In other situations, patients may be sabotaging the effectiveness of an interview for conscious reasons (i.e. malingering). In many cases, confrontations lead to the opening of new avenues of pursuit.

Example: *I've noticed that every time I ask about your appetite that we seem to get diverted onto another topic. In order to be able to help you, I need to have a better understanding of your food intake.*

I/ Echoing or Reflection
This technique involves repeating part of something that the patient just said to encourage elaboration of that area in particular.

Example:
Patient: *I played many sports in high school. I made the honor roll for three years and then dropped out.*
Interviewer: *You dropped out! What happened?*

J/ Facilitating Techniques

This is a general term outlining the techniques listed in this chapter, which encourage patients to provide you with more information.

K/ Interpretation

The term interpretation has a variety of meanings. In the context of an interview, it can be thought of as an hypothesis that the clinician suggests to the patient to explain discrepancies between observed behaviors and expressed thoughts or feelings. Interpretations are used for a variety of functions in interviews:

- To assess the degree of insight a patient possesses
- As a means of overcoming resistance to the assessment
- To facilitate the sharing of thoughts and emotional experiences

There are three components to link in an accurate interpretation:

- The thoughts, emotions or behaviors manifested
- The unconscious intent
- The reaction to the interviewer

The last item is more the domain of psychotherapy, though some interviewers include a **trial interpretation** to assess a patient's suitability for longer-term treatment. Interpretations often follow clarification and/ or confrontation.

Example:
Interviewer: *I need to double check something. You said your alcohol intake increased a lot about three months ago.* (clarification, with a closed-ended question)
Patient: *Yes, that's about right.*
Interviewer: *You said you weren't sure why, but isn't that also about the same time that your wife was promoted to CEO?* (confrontation, with a leading question)

Patient: *Yeah, pretty close.*
Interviewer: *I've noticed that every time you speak about your wife, you clench your fists and look away from me. Is it possible you're envious of her success and have turned to alcohol to numb your feelings?* (interpretation)

A complete interpretation could have occurred if it was possible to show that the patient was displaying feelings of jealousy towards the interviewer. Othmer & Othmer (1994) make the key point that an interpretation is an hypothesis, not a fact. Regardless of the elegance of your explanation, it must make sense to the patient and, for this reason, needs to be properly timed, and made in the context of a developing therapeutic alliance. Many premature, ill-timed or incorrect interpretations have led to the immediate termination of interviews and/ or psychotherapy, and can leave a lingering resentment towards the field of psychiatry.

L/ **Reiterating** or **Summarizing**
This is used to demonstrate to patients that you have heard them, and want to clarify your understanding. It also can be used to bring closure to an area of inquiry.

Example:
What I have heard you say, and please correct me if I have missed something, is that you feel awkward in social situations, fear that you might do something embarrassing and, as a result of this, chose to avoid your graduation ceremony.

M/ **Probes** or **Checks**
Probes or checks are used to obtain more information about a patient's understanding of his or her experiences. For example, asking a patient with delusions how he or she "knows" the ideas to be true is sometimes called a probe. Probes and checks can also refer to the inclusion of actual symptoms or diagnostic criteria as part of the question. The "checking of

symptoms" type of question usually follows open-ended techniques because the content of the question can influence the patient's responses (i.e. the power of suggestion).

Example:
Have you had unwanted thoughts intrude into your consciousness?

N/ Silence
Silence can be a very good facilitating technique and is particularly appropriate when you have developed some rapport with patients. Silence encourages patients to keep talking and, in this way, you have indicated that you wish to know more about the area being discussed. Generally, periods of silence should not exceed fifteen to twenty seconds and are best avoided with severely mentally ill patients.

Example:

O/ Validation
Validation establishes that the patient's feelings are reasonable and understandable given the particular circumstances.

Example: *I think anyone in your situation would feel angry.*

Interruptions
While no one enjoys being interrupted, patients will inevitably divert from the areas pertinent to the interview and, therefore, need to be refocused. Novice interviewers in particular may have a protocol that they like to follow, as they can become quickly disorganized by receiving information out of sequence. More experienced interviewers are able to "sort" the incoming information and interrupt patients less frequently. How-

ever, it is important to develop the ability to make gentle, tactful interruptions. Patients who divert you from completing a thorough interview are ultimately doing themselves a disservice. Further, patients are frequently more resilient to interruptions than we realize, and often appreciate structure. Overly talkative patients have likely been told many times about their loquaciousness, and won't take offence at a change of topic. One technique is to tell patients at the beginning of the interview that you have many areas to cover in a certain amount of time, and you may need to change the focus of the interview at times. Some supervisors are opposed to this because it may inhibit the flow of information at the start of the interview. Other techniques are:

- Empathize: *Mr. Angst, I can understand that the past month has been terrible for you. In order to more fully understand how you've been affected, I need to ask you about. . .*
- Temporize: *Your interest in infomercials is very clear, and I would like to return to them sometime later. I'd like to find out more about your family. . .*
- Redirecting: *Before my last question, I was asking you about your interest in schedules and plans. Could we return to those areas?*
- Reconnecting: *Earlier, you were telling me about your brothers and sisters. Can I ask you more about them now?*

Transitions in Topic

There is considerable ground to cover in a full interview. Patients will not provide all the information you require on each area you need to ask about on their own, even if they are health professionals themselves. You will need to observe and practice ways of making smooth transitions between topics. Othmer & Othmer (1994) outline two ways of making seamless transitions in topic:

- Cause-and-Effect Relationships: the interviewer directs the flow of information from an event or action to its psychological consequences (e.g. being fired from a job leading to poor sleep, diminished appetite, and other symptoms of depression)

- Temporal Relationships: use the time frame of reported symptoms to explore related areas (e.g. after eliciting the symptoms of an adjustment disorder, change to inquiring about alcohol intake by asking *At that time, did your pattern of alcohol intake change?*)

Echoing/ reflection also assists with effecting a smooth transition by selecting something the patient has just said and then using it as a springboard for a new line of inquiry. Complete shifts in topic can be facilitated by **reiterating/ summarizing** and then introducing the new topic. It can be helpful to announce what the new area is so the patient can shift gears and be prepared for the questions that follow.

Example: *Now that we have talked about recent events, I'd like to find out more about your employment history.*

Abrupt transitions throw off the rhythm of an interview, and often leave patients bewildered about the topic change. These types of transitions most frequently occur in three circumstances: a forgotten point from a previous section is suddenly remembered; the interviewer runs out of things to ask in a certain section; or time is running short and the interviewer is scrambling to cover a few more areas.

Othmer & Othmer (1994) indicate that abrupt transitions can be a form of cross-examination designed to throw patients off track and reveal inconsistencies in their histories. This type of interview style can be used when fabrication of symptoms is suspected (i.e. factitious disorder or malingering).

Interview Techniques

Rutter & Cox et al published a series of articles examining the use of particular techniques in psychiatric interviews. They reviewed several classic articles, but found that little systematic research had been carried out to establish the effectiveness of the methods presented in these papers. Also, the interview-related research that had been carried out only presented ways to elicit factual information. Prior to their work, no study had been conducted on the usefulness of techniques to elicit information about feelings (Rutter & Cox, 1981).

Techniques Effective in Eliciting Facts (Cox, 1981)
Non-directive (open-ended) questions are effective in encouraging patients to list their areas of difficulty. Detailed information about symptoms is typically not offered by patients, and requires systematic questioning and probing to elicit. Obtaining factual information is facilitated when the interviewer:
- Actively introduces topics and has many turns at speaking
- Asks a high number of probes/ checking questions
- Makes repeated requests for detailed information

Techniques Effective in Eliciting Feelings (Hopkinson, 1981)
Techniques which encourage patients to speak freely, and at length (i.e. open-ended questions), facilitate the expression of feelings. Closed-ended questions were seen as inhibiting emotional expression because they indicate that the interviewer has decided what is important. Eliciting feeling is facilitated when the interviewer:
- Makes direct requests for emotional reactions
- Expresses sympathy
- Uses confrontation and interpretation (when appropriate)
- Uses open-ended questions
- Reflects emotional cues

References

R. Campbell
Psychiatric Dictionary, Seventh Edition
Oxford University Press, New York, 1996

A. Cox, K. Hopkinson & M. Rutter
Psychiatric Interviewing Techniques II: Naturalistic Study: Eliciting Factual Information
British Journal of Psychiatry 138: p. 283 — 291, 1981

A. Cox, M. Rutter & D. Holbrook
Psychiatric Interviewing Techniques V: Experimental Study: Eliciting Factual Information
British Journal of Psychiatry 138: p. 29 — 37, 1981

A. Cox, D. Holbrook & M. Rutter
Psychiatric Interviewing Techniques VI: Experimental Study: Eliciting Feelings
British Journal of Psychiatry 138: p. 144 — 152, 1981

G.O. Gabbard
The Exit Line: Heightened Transference-Countertransference Manifestations at the End of The Hour
Journal of the American Psychoanalytic Association 30: p. 579 — 598, 1982

K. Hopkinson, A. Cox & M. Rutter
Psychiatric Interviewing III: Naturalistic Study: Eliciting Feelings
British Journal of Psychiatry 138: p. 406 — 415, 1981

J. Morrison
The First Interview, Revised for DSM-IV
The Guildford Press, New York, 1995

E. Othmer & S.C. Othmer
The Clinical Interview Using DSM-IV: Volume 1, The Fundamentals
American Psychiatric Press, Washington D.C., 1994

M. Rutter & A. Cox
Psychiatric Interviewing Techniques I: Methods and Measures
British Journal of Psychiatry 138: p. 273 — 282, 1981

S.C. Shea
Psychiatric Interviewing: The Art of Understanding, Second Edition
W.B. Saunders Co. Philadelphia, 1998

3/ *Identifying Features*

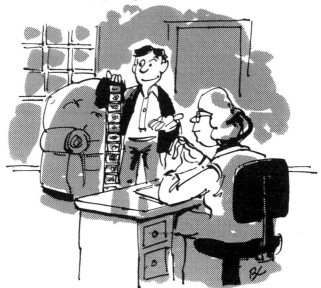

Introduction

Identifying features are the demographics of patients that help to build a mental picture of that person's unique social makeup. While this information is the first to be included in verbal and written presentations of case material, it is a matter of style as to when it is obtained. Some clinicians advocate a period of "small talk" prior to formally beginning the interview. If this can be done naturally, it is a nice way to ease into the assessment. As an alternate "icebreaker," questions can be asked about the patient's identifying features.

Gauron (1966) investigated the diagnostic decision making process in psychiatry. He reported on the various permutations of data requested in sample cases presented to the study participants (e.g. most frequently requested categories of information; categories most helpful in establishing a diagnosis, etc.). Gauron found that when psychiatrists sought information about a sample case, four of the five categories initially requested were identifying features. They were:

1. Age
2. Sex
4. Race
5. Living situation

Reason for referral was the third most requested category. Interestingly, these categories were not ultimately found to be of particular assistance in arriving at a diagnosis. For example, changing the age, gender, race or living situation of the person at the end of a hypothetical case did not cause psychiatrists to change their diagnostic impressions. Despite this, identifying features are of considerable help when clinicians are developing a mental framework on which to piece together other categories of information from the patient's history. Identifying features are:

- Name
- Age *
- Gender *
- Cultural Factors * (including race and religion)
- Marital & Parental Status *
- Occupational Status *

* These areas are presented in separate sections in this chapter.

Age

Age is one of the most significant factors governing prognosis. Two subspecialties in psychiatry have developed to deal with patients at the early and late ranges of age (Child and Geriatric Psychiatry, respectively). If patients are afflicted at an early age, they may experience an interruption in education, lose employment opportunities, and have added difficulties in finding a mate. Patients afflicted later in life are often better established, but have less "plasticity" which is important for a fuller recovery. In general, the earlier the onset of the disorder, the less optimistic is the prognosis.

Another factor to consider is the typical age of onset of a disorder. If the patient's age is outside the usual range, it may indicate the presence of a non-psychiatric cause. For example, older patients have a higher likelihood of psychiatric disorders being caused by:

- Medical conditions (e.g. hypothyroidism causing depression)
- Drug-drug interactions (older patients take more medications)
- Organic mental disorders (e.g. delirium causing behavioral disturbances)

Younger patients have a higher likelihood of substance-induced disorders (either in intoxication or withdrawal states). Typical ages of onset for major psychiatric illnesses are as follows:

Condition	Typical Age of Onset
• Schizophrenia	late teens to mid 30's
• Delusional Disorder	middle to late adulthood
• Bipolar Mood Disorder	mean is early 20's; ranges up to 50's
• Major Depression	mid 20's to mid 40's
• Dysthymia	late teens to mid 20's
• Panic Disorder	late teens and mid 30's
• Phobias	typically from childhood to mid teens
• OCD	early teens and mid 20's
• Gen. Anxiety Disorder	majority start in childhood and teens

- Somatization Disorder   before 30 (by definition of the disorder)
- Conversion Disorder   teens to late 20's
- Hypochondriasis   typically early adulthood
- Anorexia Nervosa   mid teens
- Bulimia Nervosa   late teens to early 20's
- Alcoholism   typically established by early adulthood

Each age group brings certain challenges for providing treatment. For example, younger patients who are faced with the prospect of having a life-long illness often refuse to take medication and are difficult to engage in psychotherapy. Older patients often take several medications, and considerable expertise must be employed in adding another drug to their regimen. The effectiveness of psychotherapy for the older patients may be reduced because attitudes and patterns of behavior are harder to change with age. Due to the aging population base, more attention is being given to tailoring therapies for older patients (Jeste, 1997).

Gender

Gender is a highly significant factor when considering the etiology and treatment of mental disorders. Whether differences exist because of nature (biological) or nurture (psychosocial influences), the majority of psychiatric disorders demonstrate a preponderance for one of the sexes. For example, patients suffering from eating disorders or somatization disorder are almost always women, whereas substance use disorders and paraphilias are much more common among men.

Some of the considerations in the pharmacological treatment of female patients are as follows:

- Concern during pregnancy due to the teratogenic effects of some psychiatric medications (e.g. the mood stabilizers)
- Prolactin levels can increase with use of antipsychotic medication, interfering with menses and/ or inhibiting ovulation
- The rate of growth of breast cancers can escalate with an increase in the level of prolactin

Male patients risk priapism with use of medications that cause alpha$_2$- receptor blockade (e.g. antipsychotics and antidepressants). The differential response of men and women to psychotherapeutic treatment is another area being investigated (Barbieri, 1999).

The following table summarizes gender differences in the epidemiology of psychiatric conditions (APA, 1994; Kaplan & Sadock, 1998).

Condition	Gender Ratio Male:Female
Schizophrenia	1 : 1
Delusional Disorder	1 : 1.2
Bipolar Mood Disorder	1 : 1
Major Depression	1 : 2
Dysthymia	1 : 2.5
Panic Disorder	1 : 2.5
Phobias	1 : 1.5 to 1 : 2
OCD	1 : 1
Gen. Anxiety Disorder	1 : 2
Somatization Disorder	1 : 10 or higher
Conversion Disorder	1 : 2 to 1: 10
Hypochondriasis	1 : 1
Anorexia Nervosa	1 : 10 or higher
Bulimia Nervosa	1 : 10 or higher
Alcoholism	5 : 1

Culture

More than in any other medical specialty, clinicians in psychiatry need to be aware of the significant effects that migration, religion, race, language, and family composition have on mental illness. **Social psychiatry** is concerned with how the presentation, symptoms, and management of mental illness needs to be tailored to incorporate cultural factors. Turner (1997) pointed out that immigrant groups almost universally experience higher rates of mental illness in their host (new) country, and that becoming acculturated presents particular difficulties for families composed of a number of generations. It is common, for example, for second-generation immigrants to come into conflict with their elders about the issue of maintaining traditional values versus adopting those of their new country.

While the DSM-IV is prepared and published by the **American Psychiatric Association (APA)**, it is used by clinicians for ethnically diverse populations within the United States and other countries. A number of features in the DSM-IV specifically address cultural aspects:

- A section outlining cultural factors in the description of the disorder that accompanies the diagnostic criteria; this is generally included with age and gender-specific considerations
- An outline for cultural formulation which assists clinicians in more accurately assessing the impact of an illness within the individual's cultural context (in Appendix I)
- A glossary of **culture-bound syndromes** (also in Appendix I)

A/ Diagnosis

Patients who are from a different culture than the psychiatrist evaluating them have been reported to receive a more "severe" diagnosis for their symptoms. For example, African-Americans are more likely to be diagnosed with schizophrenia than are Caucasians when presenting with similar symptoms (Price, 1985). Harrison (1988) found that rates of schizophrenia among second-generation African-Caribbeans in the UK is up to 14 times the national average.

B/ Translation & Language Interpretation

Interpretation in a medical setting is often required to go beyond translation, and needs to involve an understanding of the patient's culture. Haffner (1992) provides examples from her work with Hispanic/ Latino patients:

- A woman in labor refuses an epidural because she fears it will paralyze her, and that she needs to feel pain in order to be a real mother
- Latino women do not equate a miscarriage or stillbirth with being pregnant, and may only enumerate their successful pregnancies when asked
- Dietary restrictions during pregnancy may be difficult to encourage because of the belief that having a thin baby is unhealthy

Haffner (1992) also advises against using family members as interpreters for the following reasons:

- The interpreter is affected by what is happening to the family member and must resume his or her normal family role when the interview is over
- Physicians can place children in positions of authority which may be contrary to the family hierarchical structure
- Family members may be reluctant to describe upsetting or private symptoms in front of other family members
- Hispanic patients may feel that out of politeness they should agree with a physician's treatment plan, and may not grasp the concept of informed decision making

Medical interpretation requires a firm grasp of two languages and two cultures in order to provide the immediate, accurate, and complex information required. Poma (1987) remarked that "the language of our childhood remains the language used during times of intimacy and stress." In a detailed analysis, Price (1975) noted that interpreters obfuscated the assessment process by making the following errors: asking leading questions, distorting questions, adding information not provided by patients, deleting information that was provided, and mistranslating due to carelessness or ignorance of the English language. Price (1975) also found that the more psychotic the patient, the more likely it was that mistakes in interpretation would occur.

For the above reasons, it is strongly suggested that professional interpreters be employed whenever possible.

C/ Psychopharmacology

Pharmacokinetics is the study of the distribution and metabolism of drugs in biological systems. **Pharmocodynamics** is the study of how drugs affect biological systems which typically involves a change at receptor sites. Considerable cultural variability exists within both of these processes. Almost all psychotropic medications are metabolized by the **cytochrome P-450 (CYP)** enzyme system. These enzymes have been found to work at varying rates, thus affecting the speed with which medications are metabolized. Slow (poor) metabolizers, develop considerably higher serum drug levels than extensive (normal) metabolizers after receiving the same dose. Receptor responsiveness is another genetic factor affecting the efficacy of medications. A sample of studies reporting ethnic variation is as follows:

- A serum haloperidol level 52% higher for Asians than Caucasians for the same dose, after correcting for sex and body weight (Pi, 1989)
- Serum levels of desipramine did not vary significantly between Asians and Caucasians, though more Caucasians were found to be extensive metabolizers (Pi, 1989)

- African-American bipolar patients had higher serum lithium levels and reported more side effects compared to Caucasians (Strickland, 1995)
- Asian volunteers had higher serum levels of benzodiazepines compared to Caucasians (Lin, 1988)

A number of studies have yielded inconclusive results when examining ethnic differences. There is considerable individual variation within ethnic populations. Furthermore, non-biologic cultural factors exert powerful influences on determining the effectiveness of psychotropic medication such as: expectations, compliance, placebo effects, and side effects (Kleinman, 1988).

D/ Other Forms of Therapy
Various aspects of acculturation proceed at different rates. While immigrants may develop language skills quickly, their ideas about illness may never change. Turner (1997) reports that many immigrants make visits to traditional healers even if they are employed in health care professions. Kitron (1992) reported that therapy conducted in the patient's (but not the psychotherapist's) native tongue can assist in the process of acculturation.

E/ Religion
Gallup (1989) reports that 94% of Americans believe in God. People look to their religious leaders and literature for guidance, thus it is important to inquire about spiritual beliefs. Waldfogel (1993) points out that failure to explore a patient's religious beliefs and practices can lead to an incomplete diagnostic assessment that, in turn, overlooks options for interventions. Further, without understanding the role of religion, a clinician's own biases may lead to conflicts with patients in treatment matters. Waldfogel goes on to outline various approaches to incorporating religious factors into psychiatric evaluations. The APA (1990) has published

guidelines regarding religion and psychiatric practice:
- Information about patients' religious beliefs should be obtained
- Conflict should be handled with concern for the patient's vulnerability to the attitudes of the psychiatrist
- No practitioner should force a specific religious, antireligious or ideologic agenda on a patient
- Religious concepts or rituals should not be offered instead of accepted diagnostic and therapeutic practices

Marital & Parental Status

A patient's marital status is included when listing identifying features, though a fuller exploration is obtained in the Personal History section. This information gives an immediate picture of the patient's social supports and home environment. The presence of a spouse or partner is generally a positive indicator in psychiatry on many levels:
- It indicates a higher level of premorbid functioning
- Spouses/ partners are important sources of information
- Spouses/ partners often assist with compliance both for medications and for keeping appointments

Occupational Status

The last commonly included identifying feature is the patient's employment status. Again, while further detail is sought in the occupational history (often included as part of the Personal History), it is useful to inquire if the patient is employed, and if so, what kind of work he or she does. As with the presence of a partner or spouse, being employed is a good prognostic indicator because it demonstrates the presence of initiative, responsibility, and commitment.

Points on Technique

As presented previously, some clinicians prefer a period of informal talk before formally starting the interview. This prelude can be used to put patients at ease, find common ground or to begin collecting identifying data. The advantage to this approach is that it obtains information useful for **hypothesis generation** about the patient. Further, it can help develop rapport to assist you in asking more difficult questions. Some clinicians prefer to delay obtaining identifying information because it requires closed-ended questions, and it may be difficult to shift gears and start using open-ended questions for the History of Present Illness section. Information about identifying features can be obtained later in the interview.

Another difficulty in asking for personal information at the outset is that it has the potential to damage rapport. Elderly patients being interviewed by students may not respond well when the first question posed is *How old are you?* Many clinicians seek identifying information at the beginning of the interview, but have found less confrontational ways to word their questions. For example, the questions on the left side of the list below can be asked more delicately by using the wording on the right side.

Age
How old are you?   *What is your age?*

Religion
Are you religious?   *Do you follow a particular faith?*

Marital Status
Are you married?   *Who is at home with you?*

Culture
*Are you. . . (guess   *What is your cultural background?*
at culture)?*

Occupation
Where do you work?   *How do you support yourself?*

Example

Mr. Lo is a forty-five-year-old male of Chinese descent. He is married with two children, and works as an automotive engineer. He is a practicing Buddhist.

References

American Psychiatric Association
Guidelines Regarding Possible Conflict Between Psychiatrists' Religious Commitments and Psychiatric Practice
American Journal of Psychiatry 147: p. 542, 1990

American Psychiatric Association
Diagnostic & Statistical Manual of Mental Disorders, Fourth Edition
American Psychiatric Association, Washington, D.C., 1994

N.B. Barbieri
Psychoanalytic Contributions to the Study of Gender Issues
Canadian Journal of Psychiatry 44: p. 72 — 76, 1999

G. Gallup & J. Castelli
The People's Religion: American Faith in the 90's
Macmillan, New York, 1989

E.F. Gauron & J.K. Dickinson
Diagnostic Decision Making in Psychiatry I: Information Usage
Archives of General Psychiatry 14: p. 225 — 232, 1966

L. Haffner
Cross-Cultural Medicine: A Decade Later
Western Journal of Medicine 157: p. 255 — 259, 1992

G. Harrison
A Prospective Study of Severe Mental Disorder in Afro-Caribbean Patients
Psychological Medicine 18: p. 643 — 657, 1988

D.V. Jeste
Psychiatry of Old Age is Coming
American Journal of Psychiatry 154: p. 1356 — 1358, 1997

H.I. Kaplan & B.J. Sadock
Synopsis of Psychiatry, Eighth Edition
Williams & Wilkins, Baltimore, 1998

The Psychiatric Interview — Explained

A. Kleinman
Rethinking Psychiatry
Free Press, New York, 1988

D.G. Kitron
Transference and Countertransference Implications of Psychotherapy Conducted in a Foreign Language
Bulletin of the Menninger Clinic 56: p. 232 — 245, 1992

K.M. Lin, J.K. Lau, R. Smith, P. Phillips, E. Antal & R.E. Poland
Comparison of Alprazolam Plasma Levels in Asian and Caucasian Male Volunteers
Psychopharmacology 96: p. 365 — 369, 1988

E.H. Pi, T.K. Tran-Johnson, N.R. Walker, T.B. Cooper, R.F. Suckow & G.E. Gray
Pharmocokinetics of Desipramine in Asian and Caucasian Volunteers
Psychopharmacology Bulletin 25: p. 483 — 487, 1989

P.A. Poma
Pregnancy in Hispanic Women
Journal of the National Medical Association 79: p. 929 — 935, 1987

J. Price
Foreign Language Interpreting in Psychiatric Practice
Australian and New Zealand Journal of Psychiatry 9: p. 263 — 267, 1975

N. Price, W. Glazer & H. Morgenstern
Race and the Use of Fluphenazine Decanoate
American Journal of Psychiatry 142: p. 1491 — 1492, 1985

T.L. Strickland, K.M. Lin, P. Fu, D. Anderson, Y. Zheng
Comparison of Lithium Ratio between African American and Caucasian Bipolar Patients
Biological Psychiatry 37: p. 325 — 330, 1995

T. Turner
Ethnicity and Psychiatry
The Practitioner 241: p. 612 — 614, 1997

S. Waldfogel & P.R. Wolpe
Using Awareness of Religious Factors to Enhance Interventions in Consultation-Liaison Psychiatry
Hospital & Community Psychiatry 44: p. 473 — 477, 1993

4/ *Reason for Referral*

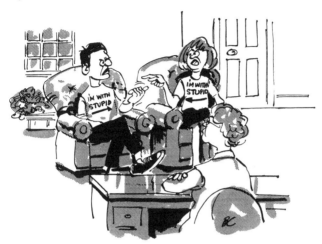

Introduction

In most situations, patients access psychiatric care after some type of screening process. In hospital settings, an assessment by an emergency physician or family doctor is the most common source of psychiatric referrals. In an emergency department, patients are asked to state the reason for their visit. Their replies are often recorded verbatim on the emergency chart. Similarly, referral letters from other sources frequently include a particular question to be addressed. The **Reason for Referral (RFR)** is also called the **Chief Complaint (CC)** or **Presenting Complaint (PC)**. Some psychiatrists avoid these terms because it may appear pejorative in the sense that patients are described as "complaining."

The main value in being aware of the RFR is that it provides essential data for hypothesis generation. Even based on a single item, experienced clinicians begin formulating ideas to assist with the interview. When the RFR is something like "racing thoughts" or "patient feels persecuted by a fountain pen," diagnostic possibilities are relatively easy to generate. Obscure RFRs (e.g. "left arm pain") are more difficult to use diagnostically at the outset (discussed below).

Hypothesis Generation With the RFR

In order to gain facility with generating hypotheses, a useful exercise is to develop a list of five possible conditions related to an individual symptom or particular complaint. On a practical level, it is difficult to work with more than five diagnoses at a time, and the vast majority of patients will have fewer than five conditions.

Two factors increase the benefit of going through this exercise: psychiatric disorders cannot be definitively diagnosed by the presence of a single symptom, and many conditions share an overlap of symptoms. For example, consider the following symptoms and their possible diagnoses:

Symptom: Paranoid Ideation
> Paranoid Schizophrenia
> Delusional Disorder, Persecutory Type
> Paranoid Personality Disorder
> Substance-Induced Psychotic Disorder (e.g. amphetamines)
> Personality Change Due to a General Medical Condition

Symptom: Grandiosity
> Manic or Hypomanic Episode
> Narcissistic Personality Disorder
> Delusional Disorder, Grandiose Type
> Paranoid Personality Disorder
> Substance Intoxication (e.g. cocaine)

A significant area of assistance with diagnostic reasoning can be found in the DSM-IV (APA, 1994), in **Appendix A, Decision Trees for Differential Diagnosis**. Here, algorithms are provided for arriving at a particular diagnosis. Of particular usefulness is the hierarchy of the questions/ probes that are used to reach a diagnostic conclusion. For example, general medical conditions and substance use must be excluded before a psychotic disorder can be diagnosed. Michael First (1995) published a book of DSM-IV-based differential diagnoses that is also a valuable resource.

Points on Technique

If the RFR is not available, asking about why a patient has come to see you is often the first question posed. The phrasing of this question can be problematic if you ask, *What brought you to the hospital today?* Some patients will say that it was an ambulance or a taxi. You can reword this question to prevent such a literal interpretation, for example:

- *What difficulties are you experiencing today?*
- *How can I be of assistance today?*

Obscure RFRs

The stated RFR may at times be unhelpful or even misleading (e.g. a complaint of left arm pain). If patients cannot provide you with information which explains the referral, ask if they understand why someone from psychiatry was asked to see them. Overly "somatic" RFRs can be due to atypical presentations of certain illnesses (i.e. depression) or are due to one of the following:

• Somatic Delusions	Fixed, false beliefs about bodily functions
• Conversion Disorder	Presence of deficits that suggest neurological or medical conditions

- Somatization Disorder — Widespread physical complaints with no demonstrable pathology

- Hypochondriasis — Persistent fears of having a serious illness

- Factitious Disorder — Self-imposed injuries or symptoms to assume the "sick role"

- Malingering — The conscious production of symptoms in order to gain some advantage (called secondary gain), such as narcotic prescriptions, absences from work, avoidance of court dates, etc.

- Culture-Bound Syndromes — Psychiatric conditions often present in ways influenced by culture; for example, depression in many parts of the world is accompanied by many physical complaints (see Appendix I in the DSM-IV)

References

American Psychiatric Association
Diagnostic & Statistical Manual of Mental Disorders, Fourth Edition
American Psychiatric Association, Washington, D.C., 1994

M.B. First, A. Frances & H.A. Pincus
DSM-IV Handbook of Differential Diagnosis
American Psychiatric Press, Inc., Washington, D.C., 1995

5/ History of the Present Illness

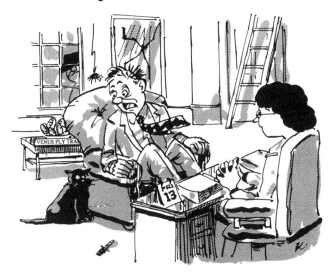

Introduction

The **History of the Present Illness (HPI)** is regarded by many psychiatrists as the most important part of the interview. Some would argue that the MSE is more important, though at least half of the MSE can be obtained in the HPI. The HPI is the section that usually takes the most time to complete.

Goals for the HPI

- Develop rapport
- Keep track of, and investigate, symptoms
- Generate and revise diagnostic hypotheses
- Record at least half of the MSE
- Keep track of cues for further exploration of facts and feelings

Structure of the HPI

The HPI can be visualized as a funnel, with open-end questions being posed at the top (beginning of the HPI) and more focused questions at the bottom (end of the HPI).

Morrison (1995), Shea (1998), and Othmer & Othmer (1994) all recommend a period of relatively unstructured time at the beginning of the HPI. Morrison (1995) advocates that a full five minutes be alloted to give patients the chance to speak freely. This increases rapport because patients will usually tell you what is troubling them the most.

One study revealed that an average of less than twenty seconds elapsed before physicians interrupted patients (Beckman & Franckel, 1984). During this initial interval, it is recommended that you use open-ended questions and facilitating techniques so that patients "tell you the story." Periods of silence greater than 15 to 20 seconds are not usually helpful.

You can certainly make interventions in the initial five minutes, but do so to keep patients talking, not to interrupt them.

Develop a Time Line — Pick a Reference Point

A technique that helps structure the HPI is to construct a time line for the patients' current difficulties. The HPI generally goes back up to one month in time. It is important to be familiar with the duration of illness stipulated in the DSM-IV when constructing a time line. For example, certain disturbances must be present for a specified time in order to meet the diagnostic criteria:

• Schizophrenia	4 weeks
• Major Depressive Episode	2 weeks
• Manic Episode	1 week
• Hypomanic Episode	4 days

The reference point that separates the present illness from the psychiatric history can be established by asking:

- *When were you last well?*
- *When were you last your usual self?*
- *At what point in time did things change for you?*

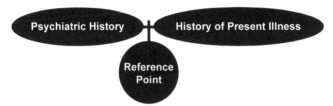

The reference point can also be determined by listening for, or asking about, a precipitant for the patient's current problems. The most common precipitants are:

- Disturbances in interpersonal relationships (DIRs)
- Substance use (e.g. intoxication or withdrawal states)
- Stopping psychiatric medications
- Starting or stopping medication used for medical illnesses
- Onset of a medical condition (e.g. hypothyroidism)

Elicit & Evaluate Symptoms

During the initial five-minute phase, some patients will give a chronological history starting at the beginning of the episode. Others will tell you about their immediate crisis. From the information patients offer, interviewers must distill out the symptoms of psychiatric disorders, and then ask about the presence of other symptoms that weren't mentioned. Next, a decision is made about whether the symptoms or complaints are of sufficient severity to be considered diagnostic criteria. Symptoms in psychiatry are explored as fully as they are in other areas of medicine. For example, a patient with chest pain would be asked about several parameters: quality, duration, radiation, frequency, severity, onset, etc.

Parameters of Psychiatric Symptoms

- Onset
- Duration
- Frequency
- Examples
- Precipitating & Ameliorating Factors
- Patient's handling of the symptoms
- Social and occupational impact of the symptoms

More About the DSM-IV

The DSM-IV uses five **axes** to make a complete diagnostic summary:

- **Axis I**: Major Psychiatric Syndromes/ Clinical Disorders
- **Axis II**: Personality Disorders, Prominent Maladaptive Personality Features, Ego Defense Mechanisms and Mental Retardation
- **Axis III**: General Medical Conditions
- **Axis IV**: Psychosocial and Environmental Problems
- **Axis V**: Global Assessment of Functioning (**GAF** Scale which ranges from 1 to 100; 0 is used when there is inadequate information)

The DSM-IV also lists severity specifiers for psychiatric conditions:

- **Mild:** Few, if any, symptoms in excess of those required to make the diagnosis are present, and symptoms result in no more than minor impairment in social or occupational functioning.
- **Moderate:** Impairment between mild and severe.
- **Severe:** Many symptoms in excess of those required to make the diagnosis, or several symptoms that are particularly severe, are present, or the symptoms result in marked impairment in social or occupational functioning.

Symptoms that cause significant distress or impairment in social, occupational, or in other important areas of functioning are considered to be diagnostic criteria. Stressors in day-to-day functioning are recorded on Axis IV. These are:

- Problems with primary support group
- Educational problems
- Occupational problems
- Housing problems
- Economic problems
- Problems with access to health care services
- Problems related to the social environment
- Problems related to interactions with the legal system/ crime

More About the MSE

The MSE is often unpopular for two reasons:

- The questions are difficult to formulate because they are not asked in other types of interviews or in other areas of medicine
- The questions appear to be of dubious relevance in making a diagnosis or developing a treatment plan

Once these two difficulties are surmounted, the MSE becomes an enjoyable and interesting aspect of interviewing. Almost half of the MSE is obtained "free" — that is through observation and by monitoring the flow of information from the first few minutes of the HPI:

"Free" Parameters	Parameters to Ask About
Level of consciousness	Orientation
Appearance	Cognitive Functioning
Behavior	Suicidal/ Homicidal Thoughts
Cooperation	Knowledge Base
Reliability	Perception
Affect	Mood
Thought Form	Thought Content

Getting to a Diagnosis

During the unstructured, "free speech" opening phase, patients will often mention a symptom, feeling, behavior or perception that corresponds to a DSM-IV diagnostic criterion. The task of the interviewer is to keep track of these pieces of information, evaluate them more fully (see parameters of psychiatric symptoms on page 56), and to ask about related symptoms of DSM-IV conditions.

Feightner (1975) & Barrows (1979) found that physicians generated their initial hypotheses in less than one minute, with an average of six conditions. At just five minutes into the interview, physicians finalized their hypotheses about which illnesses they thought the patient might have. Most of the relevant information was obtained in the first quarter of the interview.

Experienced interviewers have learned to pick up on possible diagnoses from a small number of cues. Each diagnosis has one or two particular "hallmark" or distinguishing features that are an essential component of the illness. For example, in order to diagnose depression, patients must either experience depressed mood or loss of interest or pleasure. While more criteria are needed to make this diagnosis, one or both of these symptoms must be present. In other words, the hallmark features provide a necessary, but not always sufficient, means for making a diagnosis. These hallmark symptoms are also the basis for formulating the screening questions for the **Review of Symptoms (ROS)**.

Points on Technique

A key question to ask patients during their narrative is, *What effect was this having on you?* This allows you to pose questions that either explore diagnostic criteria or determine the psychosocial changes caused by the patient's stressors.

For example:
Diagnostic Questioning
How was this affecting your. . sleep. .appetite. .energy level?

Psychosocial Questioning
How was this affecting your relationships with others?

Don't accept jargon at face value. If a patient uses a psychiatric term or diagnosis, explore what he or she means. For example, *You used the word "depression" earlier. Can you tell me how this applies to you?* Try to word the question in a way that avoids an intellectual explanation of the term (e.g. *What is your understanding of the term depression?*). Instead, get the patient to tell you about his or her own experience (e.g. *Tell me about your experience with depression*).

Summary of the HPI

In the HPI, diagnostically useful information is extracted from the patient's narrative. Diagnostic hypotheses are generated with this information, and more closed-ended methods are used for sorting out the possibilities. At the same time, questions can be asked about the psychosocial effects of the symptoms and stressors, to determine if social and/ or occupational functioning is being affected.

During the HPI, the interviewer is able to conduct at least half of the MSE because these components are obtainable from observation: level of consciousness, appearance, behavior, cooperation, reliability, affect and thought form.

In giving patients five minutes of "free speech" at the beginning of the interview, rapport develops and a therapeutic alliance is being constructed. Interviewers keeping track of key information can make smooth or seamless transitions to other areas of the interview. For example, if patients mention something about their families, this can be used to create a segue into the Family History section.

Diagnostic hypotheses must be largely formulated by the end of the HPI. It is rare to have information from the other sections of the interview (with the exception of the MSE) radically change the diagnostic possibilities that were developed during the HPI.

References

American Psychiatric Association
Diagnostic & Statistical Manual of Mental Disorders, Fourth Edition
American Psychiatric Association, Washington, D.C., 1994

H.S. Barrows
An Overview of Medical Problem Solving
University of Vermont Office of Continuing Medical Education, Burlington, Vermont, 1979

H.B. Beckman & R.M. Franckel
The Effect of Physician Behavior on the Collection of Data
Annals of Internal Medicine 101: p. 692 — 696, 1984

J.W. Feightner, G.R. Norman, H.S. Barrows & V.R. Neufeld
A Comparison of the Clinical Methods of Primary and Secondary Care Physicians
Association of American Medical Colleges, Washington D.C., 1975

J. Morrison
The First Interview, Revised for DSM-IV
The Guildford Press, New York, 1995

E. Othmer & S.C. Othmer
The Clinical Interview Using DSM-IV: Volume 1, The Fundamentals
American Psychiatric Press, Washington D.C., 1994

S.C. Shea
Psychiatric Interviewing: The Art of Understanding, Second Edition
W.B. Saunders Co. Philadelphia, 1998

6/ *Psychiatric History*

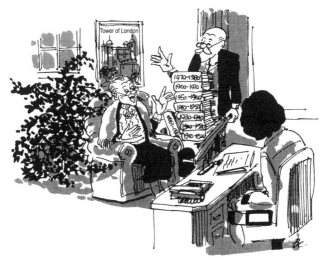

Introduction

Once the HPI is completed, the next section of the interview focuses on developing an understanding of the patient's psychiatric difficulties across his or her entire lifespan. This section is the **Psychiatric History**, and is often referred to as the **Past Psychiatric History** (even though this is redundant — all history is in the past), abbreviated as **PPH**.

Goals for the PPH

- Develop a time line for the duration of the patient's illness
- Determine the course and severity of the disorder
- Formulate an understanding of the predisposing, precipitating, perpetuating, and protective factors affecting the condition
- Obtain information about hospitalizations

- Get the details about which treatments have been tried and their effectiveness (for psychotherapy and medication)
- Assess insight and judgment

Completing the Time Line

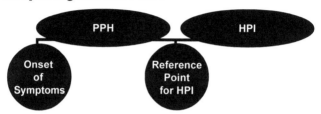

In the PPH, the focus shifts to eliciting a history of the entire duration of the patient's illness. Using the time line developed for the HPI, the emphasis is now on the events leading up to the reference point. The PPH can be obtained in chronological order, with emphasis on the following information:

- Age of onset (discussed in the Identifying Features Chapter)
- Level of functioning prior to the onset of the illness
- Level of functioning between episodes of the illness
- Number of episodes of the illness
- Number of hospitalizations (which can be used as an indicator of the severity of the illness)

The psychiatric history can be plotted on a simple graph. The Y axis can represent the presence or severity of symptoms (e.g. none, some, moderate, severe) or level of functioning (good, fair, poor). The X axis is time and starts with the onset of the first episode of the illness.

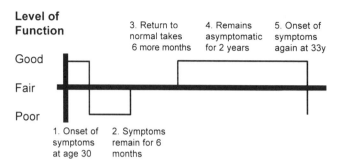

Level of Function

- Good
- Fair
- Poor

3. Return to normal takes 6 more months
4. Remains asymptomatic for 2 years
5. Onset of symptoms again at 33y
1. Onset of symptoms at age 30
2. Symptoms remain for 6 months

On pages 9 & 10, the **biopsychosocial approach** to understanding psychiatric illness was introduced, complete with a grid. An example of information from the PPH listed in grid form for a patient suffering from depression is as follows:

	Biological	**Social**	**Psychological**
Predisposing	genetic loading for depression (strong family history)	awkward and shy around others	loss of mother when the patient was age 9
Precipitating	use of street drugs (cocaine and amphetamines)	break-up of long-term relationship	failed university exams and other academic problems
Perpetuating	unrecognized hypothyroidism	few friends or social supports available	low esteem; reluctant to attempt new course at university
Protective	general health is good; will avoid using street drugs in the future	has assistance program available through work	above-average intelligence; diversified interests

Course & Severity of An Illness

After establishing the patient's age and premorbid level of functioning at the onset of the disorder, use open-ended techniques to facilitate a narrative summary about the illness. You are particularly interested in the impact the illness has made on the patient, and those close to him or her. Questions about the overall severity of the illness can be posed as follows:

- *What opportunities were lost because of the illness?*
- *How is the patient different as a result of the illness?*
- *How does the patient cope?*

The course of the entire illness can be illustrated as on page 63. Individual episodes can be recorded as follows:

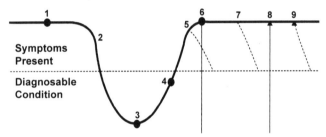

Key

1. Period of normal or usual functioning
2. **Onset** of symptoms
3. Condition is at its most severe; treatment is sought
4. **Response** to treatment occurs
5. **Remission** — a return of symptoms or increase in symptom severity before a complete recovery from the illness
6. **Recovery** — a return to the premorbid level of functioning
7. **Relapse** — a return of symptoms or increase in symptom severity after there has been complete recovery from the illness

8. Continuation of recovery — an arbitrarily defined period of time, often from six months to one year, where various forms of treatment can be discontinued
9. **Recurrence** — a completely new episode of the illness

Hospitalizations

In general, the greater the number of hospitalizations a patient has had, the more serious is the severity. Information about previous inpatient stays is a very important guide for future treatment plans. While you would like to know the details of each hospitalization, some patients have such an extensive psychiatric history that this is impractical to obtain (even if the patient can recall the details). In these situations, the following information is of greatest use:

*   The total number of hospitalizations
*   The date, duration, and reasons for the first hospitalization
*   The date, duration, and reasons for the most recent hospitalization
*   The presence of themes or patterns for readmission (e.g. medication non-compliance, street drug use, etc.)

The number of hospitalizations can be misleading because patients are often encouraged to be admitted, but refuse to do so. It is often useful to ask if anyone suggested the patient be admitted at some point in the past. Alternatively, some patients are admitted frequently for social reasons, making their illnesses appear spuriously severe.

Treatment History

The types of treatment a patient has previously received is of vital importance in developing a treatment plan. After you have gained an understanding of the course and severity of the patient's condition, ask about past (and current) treatment. Questions about treatment can be posed as follows:

- *What type of help did you receive in the past?*
- *How was your condition managed previously?*
- *Has anything made a difference in how you're feeling?*

Treatment in psychiatry generally consists of psychotherapy, pharmacotherapy, and other.

Psychotherapy Questions
- Type & duration of therapy
- Intensity of therapy (number of sessions per week or month)
- Termination of therapy (mutual, patient stopped, etc.)
- Results of therapy (a useful question to ask is, *What did you learn about yourself in therapy?*)

Pharmacotherapy Questions
- Type of medications used, dosages, and duration of treatment
- Benefits of medication (if any)
- Side effects (often a means of identifying compliance)
- Compliance with, and termination of, medication usage

Other Treatments
- Electroconvulsive Therapy (ECT)
- Community Supports
- Vocational Rehabilitation
- Religious Counseling

Current Treatment

Some interviewers ask about current treatment in the HPI, PPH or in the Medical History section. Regardless of where you ask, be sure to inquire about current psychotherapy, use of psychiatric medications, and a list of all those involved in providing assistance to the patient.

Insight & Judgment

Insight and judgment are assessed as parts of the MSE. The PPH provides an excellent opportunity to gauge these areas by looking at the patient's awareness of his or her illness, and the actions taken to seek help when that person was ill.

Insight refers to the knowledge and awareness of the parameters involved in an event, process or decision. In mental health, this term is used to describe:
- The awareness of having an illness
- An understanding of the factors contributing to, and maintaining the illness
- An appreciation that various signs and symptoms are part of a psychiatric condition

Judgment is the opinion or conclusion arrived at by a patient, and generally refers to:
- A decision
- Whether or not a certain action took place, and why
- Weighing the consequences of doing something or not doing something

Intact insight and judgment are crucial factors in making successful therapeutic interventions and are key determinants of the patient's prognosis.

References

D.J. Robinson
Brain Calipers: The Comprehensive Psychiatric Mental Status Examination
Rapid Psychler Press, Port Huron, Michigan, 1997

D.J. Robinson
Psychiatric Mnemonics & Clinical Guides, Second Edition
Rapid Psychler Press, Port Huron, Michigan, 1998

7/ Medical History

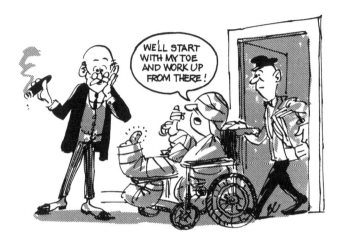

Introduction

Studies conducted by Langsley (1982 & 1988) elucidated the core skills and knowledge that define a specialist in psychiatry. The aggregate #1 ranked item on the knowledge scale was the ability to distinguish between a medical (**organic**) and a psychiatric (**functional**) disorder. The ability to make this distinction is so important that a subspecialty of psychiatry, called **Consultation-Liaison (C-L)**, focuses on the interface between medical and psychiatric disorders. Furthermore, this is why psychiatrists must complete general medical training before embarking on specialty training.

The **Medical History (MedHx)** is the section of the interview where inquiries are made about the presence of physical problems and the treatment being given for these conditions.

Goals for the MedHx

- Enumerate the patient's medical and surgical illnesses
- Ascertain which illnesses are currently active, and determine the course and severity of these conditions
- Get a list of the patient's medications
- Ask about allergies, reactions to medications, side-effects, and if the person wears a Medic-Alert bracelet or chain
- Screen for medical conditions that are of particular relevance to psychiatry, or if time permits, conduct a general medical review of systems

Medical Illness in Psychiatric Patients

Anfinson (1992) reported that up to 80% of psychiatric inpatients had significant physical illnesses. Koryani (1979) found that in almost half of psychiatric inpatients, family physicians were unaware of their patients' medical illnesses. In two-thirds of cases, the medical illness was deemed to significantly affect the psychiatric illness and, in one-fifth of cases, it was deemed to be the cause. Anfinson (1992) reminds us that the history is the most useful means for diagnosing physical conditions. This is followed by the physical exam and then by lab testing. The following battery detects over 90% of medical disorders: history, physical and neurological examinations; SMA-34 blood chemistry, EKG, urinalysis, and sleep-deprived EEG.

The Relationship Between Physical and Psychiatric Illnesses

There are four sets of interactions to consider when patients have both a medical and psychiatric illness (**comorbidity**):
- Psychiatric Disorders Affecting Medical Illnesses
- Psychiatric Treatment Affecting Medical Illnesses
- Medical Illnesses Affecting Psychiatric Disorders
- Medical Treatment Affecting Psychiatric Conditions

The Effects of Psychiatric Comorbidity

It has been shown that patients who suffer from both physical and psychiatric illnesses incur greater health costs and have a less optimistic prognosis for their conditions (Saravay, 1994). An unfortunate relationship between physical and psychiatric conditions can exist in that they perpetuate one another (described above and below).

Possible Medical Complications Resulting from Psychiatric Disorders

Schizophrenia
- Respiratory disorders and lung cancer from cigarette smoking
- Coronary artery disease due to diet, obesity, lack of exercise, etc.
- Dental caries from anticholinergic side-effects of medication

Mood Disorders
- Infections from impaired immune function during depression
- Obesity from hyperphagia, carbohydrate craving during certain types of depressive episodes, and antidepressant side-effects

Bulimia Nervosa
- Electrolyte disturbances, dehydration, alkalosis
- Mallory-Weiss tears due to repeated vomiting

Anorexia Nervosa
- The most worrisome complications are cardiac: arrhythmias, bradycardia, hypotension, and congestive heart failure
- Kidney stones; osteoporosis; amenorrhea; hypercortisolemia

Points on Technique

It is usually easy to make the transition from PPH to the MedHx. In order to let the patient know you are shifting gears, you can announce your new area of inquiry by saying something like, *At this point, I'd like to ask about your physical health.* The opening question can be open-ended, as in other sections of the interview:

- *Do you have any medical problems?*
- *Have you had any illness or operations before?*
- *Do you see your family doctor or a specialist on a regular basis for a particular problem?*

Ideally you would like to catalog the entire medical history, but some patients have several conditions, or have such a convoluted history that it is not practical to record it all. In these situations, focus on:

- The current illnesses and treatments
- The most serious illnesses
- The illness with the most relevance to psychiatry

It is important to record the MedHx relatively early in the interview, because you want to know as soon as possible if there might be an "organic" cause that either started or is perpetuating a psychiatric condition. **Organic** in this capacity means the effects of a medical illness or a substance (either a street drug or a prescribed medication). Organic factors cause psychiatric disorders that are indistinguishable from the "real thing" (often called **primary psychiatric disorders**). For this reason, it is important to go through the diagnostic exercise of considering all possible etiologies for a patient's illness.

Some clinicians include a medical review of systems as part of the MedHx, others ask about this information when the physical examination is conducted.

Caveats

Some patients do not think that their medical histories are particularly relevant and will be reluctant to share this information. Some patients legitimately forget their medical histories. The stress of their current situation, and cognitive difficulties caused either by illness or psychiatric medications, can impair recall. For this reason, check the hospital record, the family physician's office, and with family members as sources of collateral information. Patients frequently do not know the generic or trade names of their medications, just the color, size, and shape. The Physician's Desk Reference (**PDR** in the U.S.) and the Compendium of Pharmaceutical Specialties (**CPS** in Canada) have a photographic index for identifying medication. The current medication regimen can also be obtained through the family doctor or pharmacy. Don't forget to ask about medications that were recently discontinued, and if the dosages were recently changed.

References

T.J. Anfinson & R.G. Kathol
Screening Laboratory Evaluation in Psychiatric Patients: A Review
General Hospital Psychiatry 14: p. 2481 — 257, 1992

E.K. Koryani
Morbidity and Rate of Undiagnosed Physical Illness in a Psychiatric Population
Archives of General Psychiatry 36: p. 414 — 419, 1979

D.G. Langsley & M.H. Hollender
The Definition of a Psychiatrist
American Journal of Psychiatry 139: p. 81 — 85, 1982

D.G. Langsley & J. Yager
The Definition of a Psychiatrist: Eight Years Later
American Journal of Psychiatry 145: p. 469 — 475, 1988

S.M. Saravay & M. Lavin
Psychiatric Comorbidity and Length of Stay in the General Hospital: A Critical Review of Outcome Studies
Psychosomatics 35(3): p. 233 — 252, 1994

8/ *Substance Use History*

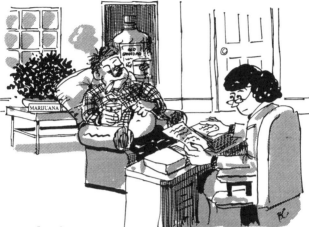

Introduction

The **history of psychoactive substance use (SubHx)** is a crucial area to ask about in interviews, and a fascinating area for psychiatric research. Psychiatric conditions can be perfectly mimicked by the use of some substances, providing a key area for investigation into the neurochemical basis of mental illness. The presence of substance abuse obscures an accurate diagnostic assessment. The DSM-IV criteria for most major clinical disorders contain an exclusionary statement that a diagnosis cannot be made if symptoms are due to the effects of a substance or a general medical condition. Clinicians vary in their opinions on how long a period of abstinence is required before psychiatric symptoms can be considered as due to a primary illness instead of a substance use. The DSM-IV considers early remission to begin one month after the time that no criteria are met for substance abuse or dependence (outlined below). Substance use is universally considered to

be a poor prognostic indicator. It is associated with:
- Poorer response to treatment
- Poorer compliance with treatment
- An increase in the number, and severity of, recurrences

There is a high degree of reciprocity between substance misuse and psychiatric illness. About 75% of men and 65% of women who had substance-related diagnoses also met the criteria for other psychiatric conditions (Warner, 1995).

Goals for the SubHx
- Determine the consumption pattern of psychoactive substances
- Screen for the presence of substance misuse
- Screen for the use of substances that are impairing social or occupational functioning and causing medical, legal or psychological problems; obtain information about the following parameters of use:

"DRAPE"

Duration of use
Route (inhaled, ingested, snorted, injected)
Amount
Pattern of use (binge, daily, solitary, etc.)
Effects (direct, adverse, etc.)

The Spectrum of Substance-Related Problems
Substance-Related Disorders have an incredible impact on society. Up to 1 in 8 people meet the diagnostic criteria for a substance-related condition. This ranks substance use disorders as being among the most prevalent of psychiatric conditions, and highlights the need for thorough assessments. Mintz (1980) found that unaddressed problems go unreported in interviews. Use of substances can have deleterious effects

in a number of aspects of patients' lives. The major areas and some typical problems are listed below:

- Family Problems
- Social Functioning
- Physical Health Problems
- Psychological Health Problems
- Legal Difficulties
- Occupational Functioning

Substance-Related Disorders

The DSM-IV defines various diagnoses based on intoxication and withdrawal for each drug of abuse. Additionally, two use-related disorders are recognized, **Substance Abuse** and **Substance Dependence**.

Substance Abuse
"HELP"

Hazardous circumstances do not deter substance use

Evasion of obligations due to substance use

Legal difficulties caused by use of substance

Problems (social and interpersonal) develop due to use

Substance Dependence
"ROLAID PUPILS"

Relief of withdrawal symptoms with substance use
(withdrawal criterion #2)

Occupational/ social/ recreational activities are given up or reduced

Larger amounts are taken than intended

Awareness of problems related to substance use

Increased amounts are needed to achieve the same effect
(tolerance criterion #1)

Diminished effect with use of the same amount
(tolerance criterion #2)

Persistent desire to cut down or control use
Unsuccessful efforts to cut down or control use
Personal problems (social and interpersonal) due to use
Investment of time in substance-related activity is considerable
Longer duration of use than initially intended
Symptoms of withdrawal occur (withdrawal criterion #1)

- The signs and symptoms of dependence or abuse must be present within the same 12-month period to make the diagnosis
- Dependence is a more serious condition than abuse; if the criteria for dependence have been met, abuse is not diagnosed

Cues to the Presence of Substance Misuse

Difficulties often start first within the family, and go on to affect the other areas of the patient's life (listed on page 75). Thus, asking questions about the state of the patient's current relationships with significant others indirectly screens for the possibility of substance misuse. In some situations, information about substance use may only be available from family members, friends, co-workers, etc. Collateral information is available from the family doctor, hospital chart, etc. Clearly, consent is required before speaking with others.

Unexplained laboratory and physical findings also provide valuable clues about substance use such as: trauma, infections, biochemical abnormalities, hematologic abnormalities, weight loss, insomnia, etc. This is particularly true for prolonged alcohol abuse because it affects the brain, blood cells, and several internal organs.

Experienced interviewers are often able to pick up subtle process signs that reveal possible difficulties with substances:
- Looking away from the interviewer when asked questions

- A sudden shift in body posture
- Change in tone of voice
- Anxiety, fidgetiness
- Changes in facial expression
- Hesitation

There are often also typical replies to initial screening questions that indicate the presence of a problem. For example, when asking about alcohol consumption, a cue to misuse might be revealed by the following answers:

- *I never drink on Sundays.*
- *I only drink beer.*
- *My doctor says red wine with dinner is good for me.*

In general, evasive answers, alibis, excuses, and rationalizations are indications of substance use problems.

Points on Technique

In the scheme outlined in this text, questions about substance use fall at about the halfway point in the interview. It often takes this amount of time to develop enough of a rapport with patients to ask about this sensitive area. Many interviewers find it helpful to ask about substance use as a subsection of the medical history. The transition between asking about physical problems and prescription medications to lifestyle and substance use can usually be made smoothly. If either you or the patient are uncomfortable with questions about substance use at this point in time, the SubHx can be integrated with the Personal History, which occurs later in the interview. You can also begin asking about substance use after the MedHx, and if the patient reacts negatively, resume questioning at the end of the Personal History.

Questions about substance use, along with sexuality and suicidal intent, pose the greatest challenges for novice interviewers. To a large extent, this is because patients have difficulty discussing these areas. Lucas (1977) found that patients were more accurate about their alcohol consumption when responding to a computer questionnaire than speaking with an interviewer. Wilson (1981) found that administering a standard form (diagnostic test) to patients was more valuable in obtaining a substance use history than was a free-form interview.

The substance use history can begin with questions about prescription medications (e.g. for pain control) or legal substances (e.g. nicotine and caffeine). A progression to questions about harder drugs (e.g. alcohol) and illicit substances can then follow. Typically, marijuana is the first recreational drug asked about because its use is relatively common, and a reasonable argument can be made for its benign effects. This is one area of the interview where leading questions can help. Rather than asking if recreational drugs are used, many clinicians phrase initial questions to assume the person uses substances, and ask how much is consumed. For example:

- *How much alcohol would you say you drink in a (day, week, month)?*
- *How much experimentation did you do with recreational drugs?*

A list of substances which can be abused are contained in the following mnemonic:

Drugs of Abuse
"COCAINE CHOPS"

Cocaine
Opioids
Cannabis

Amphetamines
Inhalants & Solvents
Nicotine
Ethanol & Non-beverage alcohol

Caffeine
Hallucinogens
Other
PCP — phencyclidine
Sedative-hypnotics

Use of leading questions is fairly common and often successful. Clearly you have to use this method with discretion, as some people will be offended at the insinuation that they use or have used substances.

Another approach is to give a preamble indicating that taking a substance history is very important to your overall understanding of the person, and that these are standard questions you ask. For example:
Now that I have asked about your medical health, I'd like to ask you some questions about your lifestyle and habits. I understand that asking questions about these areas makes some people uncomfortable. However, I am thorough, and in an interview it is very important for me to get a complete picture of you and your situation, which includes this part of your life. For instance, many people consume alcohol or tobacco — do you use either of these at times?

It is important to emphasize to patients that you are interested in this area for medical reasons, not on legal or ethical grounds. Many patients are reluctant to share this information because it becomes part of their medical record, and they don't want this information to be "used against them" at a future time (e.g. for prospective employers or in court). For this reason, you need to be familiar with the legal practices about confidentiality in your area. Asking about substance use in a straight forward, non-judgmental manner indicates to patients that you are familiar with various patterns of misuse, and are comfortable in hearing what they have to say.

References

American Psychiatric Association
Diagnostic and Statistical Manual of Mental Disorders, Fourth Edition
American Psychiatric Association, Washington D.C., 1994

R.F. Klein, M. Friedman-Campbell & R.V. Tocco
History Taking and Substance Abuse Counseling with the Pregnant Patient
Clinical Obstetrics and Gynecology 36: p. 338 — 346, 1993

R.W. Lucas, P.J. Mullin, C.B.X. Luna et al
Psychiatrists and a Computer as Interrogators of Patients With Alcohol-Related Illnesses
British Journal of Psychiatry 131: p. 160 — 167, 1977

J. Mintz, P. Christoph, C. O'Brien et al
The Impact of the Interview Method on Reported Symptoms of Narcotic Addicts
International Journal of Addiction 15: p. 597 — 604, 1980

R.A. Ruden, with M. Byalick
The Craving Brain
Harper Collins, New York, 1997

I. Stolerman
Drugs of Abuse: Behavior Principles, Methods and Terms
Trends in Pharmacological Science 13: p. 170 — 176 , 1992

L.A. Warner, R.C. Kessler, M. Hughes, J.C. Anthony & C.B. Nelson
Prevalence and Correlates of Drug Use and Dependency in the United States: Results From the National Comorbidity Survey
Archives of General Psychiatry 52: p. 219 — 229, 1995

J.R. Weinberg
Interview Techniques for Diagnosing Alcoholism
American Family Physician 9: p. 107 — 115, 1974

9/ *Family History*

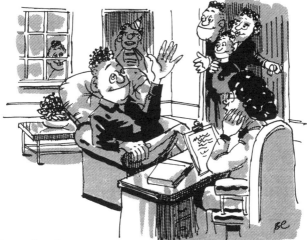

Introduction

The **Family History (FamHx)** along with the Personal History (PersHx) are two "softer" areas of the interview in terms of establishing a diagnosis. While these sections certainly can make a contribution to hypothesis generation and testing, they are typically more useful for establishing the psychosocial factors that have shaped patients' lives. In time-limited situations, the FamHx can be minimized or deferred. There is a strategic benefit to asking about the FamHx ahead of the PersHx (discussed in the next chapter).

Goals for the FamHx

- Generate a list of immediate family members and obtain key psychosocial information about each of them
- Catalog the presence of mental illness in the extended family

- Determine if there are psychiatric illnesses that cluster in family members to whom patients are genetically related
- Determine if neurologic or serious medical illnesses cluster in family members to whom patients are genetically related

There is an arbitrary dividing line between what is considered to be in the domain of FamHX and PersHx. The approach outlined here is to include information about immediate and extended family members in the FamHx (family of origin), leaving the PersHx to focus on the patient and the patient's family of creation.

Points on Technique

As with other transitions during the interview, it may help to announce to patients that you'd like to shift the focus to ask questions about their family background. This can be done in an open-ended manner by asking patients to describe their immediate and extended families of origin. For extended family members (i.e. grandparents, great aunts, aunts, great uncles, uncles, cousins), or those that the patient "is related to by blood" ask about the following:

- The presence of psychiatric symptoms or unusual behaviors
- Known psychiatric disorders and treatments
- Significant medical and neurologic illnesses
- The presence of especially significant alliances within the family

The DSM was first published in 1952 by the APA. One of the aims of this publication was to help standardize descriptive psychopathology and diagnostic practices. For example, terms such as paranoia, schizophrenia, and neurosis have historically been used to describe a wide variety of illnesses. Psychiatrists in various centers, cities, and countries employed such different methods that a diagnosis made in one place often meant little to clinicians elsewhere. In generations past, many people did not have the opportunity to see a psychiatrist, or chose not to for personal or family reasons. It is important to take these factors into account in the FamHx. Furthermore, there were few effective treatments, so it is difficult to discern what conditions may have been present from a description of the remedies that were used. A list of possible psychosocial features indicating that a relative from previous generations suffered from a psychiatric condition is as follows:

- Substance dependence (usually alcohol)
- Living in isolation (either a personal or family preference)
- Completed or attempted suicide
- Eccentric behavior
- Unexplained changes in location (e.g. immigration)
- "Nervous breakdowns" or episodes of decompensation

More information is sought about immediate family members, such as the following (which may not be obtainable in the first interview):

- Composition of the family (including birth order of siblings)
- Understanding the dynamics of the family (e.g. child-centered, parent-centered, parent-directed, etc.)
- Marital status, family size, and sexual orientation of siblings
- Type of relationship each family member had with the patient (e.g. close, distant, changed over time, etc.)
- Level of education and occupation for each member
- The presence of psychiatric symptoms or unusual behaviors
- Known psychiatric disorders or treatments
- Significant medical and neurologic illnesses
- Significant events within the family (accidents, lottery prizes, etc.)

If possible, it is very helpful to get patients to "tell you stories" or give examples to describe family members. One advantage of asking open-ended questions is that the order in which family members are listed can reveal the presence of a conflict. Often the family member involved in a difficult situation with the patient is listed last, or not at all.

Estimated Rates of the Genetic Contribution to Psychiatric Disorders

Condition	Lifetime Prevalence in the Gen. Population	Lifetime Risk with an Affected First Degree Relative
Schizophrenia	1%	8 — 47%
Delusional Disorder	0.03%	?
Bipolar Mood Disorder	1%	8 — 75%
Major Depression	15%	15 — 50%
Dysthymia	5%	?
Panic Disorder	4%	16 — 32%
Phobias	10%	66 — 75%
OCD	3%	35%
Generalized Anxiety Dis.	5%	15 — 50%
Somatization Disorder	0.5%	10 — 29%
Conversion Disorder	0.02%	?
Hypochondriasis	4%	?
Anorexia Nervosa	1%	5%
Bulimia Nervosa	2%	?
Alcoholism	10%	30 — 40%

(Source: Kaplan & Sadock, 1998)

The rates in the right column vary with the identity of the affected individual. Rates are highest for monozygotic twins, and decrease as there is less of a genetic overlap. Family history can be important in helping sort out likely diagnoses in situations where there is considerable overlap in symptoms (e.g. acute psychosis vs. mania; negative symptoms in schizophrenia vs. depression).

Psychosocial factors within families have an influence on potential psychiatric conditions. Leman (1998) outlines typical personality traits based on birth order:

- Oldest: takes charge, aggressive, perfectionistic, organized
- Middle: compromising, diplomatic, secretive, social lion
- Youngest: charming, attention seeking, uncomplicated

There is some evidence to show that there is a higher incidence of obsessive-compulsive personality disorder in the eldest child (Kaplan & Sadock, 1998).

References

H.I. Kaplan & B.J. Sadock
Synopsis of Psychiatry, Eighth Edition
Williams & Wilkins, Baltimore, 1998

K. Leman
The New Birth Order Book
Baker Book House Co., Grand Rapids, MI, 1998

10/ Personal History

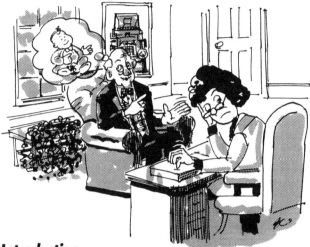

Introduction

The **Personal History (PersHx)** focuses on psychosocial development and the patient's adaptation to social and occupational roles (e.g. as a member of a family, a member of society in general, etc.). The FamHx can record information about the patient's family of origin. The PersHx collects information about the patient's development, first as part of a family, and then in areas of individuation. Many topics can easily be shifted between the FamHx and PersHx based on style, patient's replies, level of interest, etc.

Goals for the PersHx

Some of the separate sections listed in the Anatomy of the Psychiatric Interview section on pages 8 & 9 can be subsumed under the PersHx (specifically items F, G & H). A complete PersHx involves the following areas:

- Developmental History
- Child & Adolescent Psychiatric Disorders
- Social & Sexual History
- Abuse History
- Legal History
- Military History
- Obstetrical History
- Occupational/ Educational History

Points on Technique

The PersHx section is one of the easiest parts of the interview to introduce. If you have taken the FamHx first, questions centering on the patient's developmental history can usually be seamlessly integrated. If the PersHx is being asked about before the FamHx, it can be introduced as follows:

Up until now, I've been asking you a lot of questions about recent events, symptoms, medical problems, and personal habits. I'd like to change the focus at this point to find out more about you as a person and the important factors that have shaped your life. Going right back to your birth, can you tell me about your background and early years?

During the initial unstructured part of the HPI, patients are very likely to mention important parts of the PersHx. This information can be used to make a smooth transition into the PersHx, for example:

At the beginning of the interview, you were telling me about your difficulties at work and with your spouse. At this point, I'd like to return to these areas, but in order for me to have an understanding of the whole situation, I'd like to get some information about your early years and development.

Many clinicians try to keep patients focused on matters relevant to the section of the interview being asked about at a certain point in time. For example, a patient who starts giving information about her high school reunion during the MedHx can be told that such information is important, but will be requested later in the interview. The interviewer then gently directs the patient back to the present area of inquiry. By reintroducing the previously interrupted topics, patients know that you've listened to them and care about what they have to say. The PersHx falls well into the interview, and hopefully, by this point your empathic comments and/ or actions have helped establish a good working rapport with patients. There are particularly sensitive areas that still require exploration, and will be much less awkward if patients feel comfortable with you. These areas are:

*   The substance use history (if this section was deferred from being taken at the end of the MedHx)
*   A sexual history (p. 90)
*   Episodes of sexual, physical or emotional abuse (p. 93)
*   Suicidal or homicidal ideation (Appendix A)

There is a strategic advantage to taking the FamHx prior to the PersHx. The PersHx is generally obtained in chronological order which, at its conclusion, brings you right back to the information you were collecting in the HPI. This allows you to direct further inquiries into three key areas:

*   Asking about symptoms or related matters that you omitted when initially taking the HPI
*   Reiterating key symptoms to introduce the MSE (for example, if patients complain about poor memory or concentration, this is a great opportunity to formally test these areas and create a smooth transition to other areas that require investigation)
*   Reiterating key symptoms and conducting a psychiatric **Review of Symptoms (ROS)** to further confirm your hypothesis testing by asking about conditions related to those in your differential diagnosis (this is covered in Chapter 11 on p. 97)

The Developmental History

Questions about development can be divided into discrete time periods, with major points of emphasis as follows:

Pre & Postnatal Development
- Birthplace (e.g. home vs. hospital; foreign country, etc.)
- Gestational age at delivery
- Complications at delivery (low APGAR, birth anoxia, etc.)
- Postnatal complications (jaundice, infections, etc.)
- mother's health pre-, peri- and postnatally (e.g. anemia, pre-eclampsia, post-partum blues/ depression, etc.)
- Preparedness of family for patient's birth (planned, un-planned, stability of parents' relationship, etc.)

Early Childhood
- Developmental milestones achieved

3 months —	reaches for object
6 months —	single syllable words
9 months —	manipulates objects with hands
12 months —	walking; able to say one or two words; cooperates with dressing
24 months —	2 word phrases
36 months —	toilet training; consolidation of gender

- Age appropriate entry into the school system
- Problems at school (e.g. repeated grade, special education classes, truancy problems, discipline problems, etc.)
- Evaluation by a child psychiatrist (problems referred for, results of the assessment, treatment instituted)
- Administration of a structured assessment by a psychologist or other health care professional (tests are available for: intellectual ability, developmental level, achievement, adaptive behavior, projective testing, personality testing, and neuropsychiatric testing)
- Diagnosis made of a childhood psychiatric disorder

Later Childhood
- Sociability ("best" friend, groups of friends, loner, etc.)
- Interests & hobbies (e.g. sports, music, art, etc.)
- Strengths & weaknesses at school; grades
- Stability of family (e.g. separations, divorce, etc.)
- Stability of location (frequency of moves)

Social History

Some questions about social history were outlined in the previous section. As children, many people are encouraged to play sports or join organizations. The more useful aspects of the social history occur in high school and later when individuals have stronger preferences and more of an ability to control their time. In general, you are interested in getting information about membership in organizations and close relationships. It is usually easier to ask about the former first, and then about more intimate relationships. Key aspects of the social history are as follows:
- Age the person started dating
- Parental/ family attitude to dating
- Number of serious relationships, marital status, etc.
- Current social supports
- Role that religion plays/played in social development
- Description of typical patterns in past relationships
- Description of the current relationship —
  - Duration and intensity
  - What attracted the person to his or her significant other?
  - Status (e.g. together, separated, fighting, getting along, etc.)

Sexual History

Avoidance of the sexual history is an unfortunate, but not uncommon aspect of interviewing:

- Matthews (1989) found that 47% of patients had never had their family physicians ask about sexual relationships
- Lewis (1987) discovered that only 10% of family physicians obtained enough of a sexual history to determine HIV risk factors
- Ende (1984) noted that 91% of patients considered it appropriate that physicians take a sexual history
- Ende (1984) determined that only about 10% of patients were assertive enough to request help about a sexual matter

There are several barriers to taking a sexual history which can be divided into clinician and patient factors:

Clinician Factors
- Lack of time in the interview

- Fear of being intrusive or voyeuristic

- View training as inadequate to ask typical questions

- Fear of becoming attracted to, or viewed as being attracted to, patients

- Uncomfortable with where to turn for resources for patients

Patient Factors
- Age, cultural, gender or value differences with the clincian
- Patients may misconstrue questions as an invitation
- Perpetrators of sexual abuse or unsafe sexual practices may cause interviewer discomfort
- Presence of a third party can interfere with the assessment, especially with adolescents
- Concerns about confidentiality, particularly for abuse, abortion, or sexually transmitted diseases

Volmer (1989) found that students who had discussed a personal matter with a physician were more comfortable in taking a sexual history. Students are more comfortable when a scripted set of sexual history questions is provided for them. They are also more comfortable after having had the chance to watch a supervisor take a sexual history. Thorough training for sexual history taking can involve: formal seminars, group discussion, video taping, role playing, personal awareness groups, development of a sexual questionnaire, and meeting people from the community who are HIV positive.

Points on Technique
Risen (1995) echoes the sentiments of many mental health professionals in reporting that discussing sexual issues with patients engenders a degree of anxiety and a lack of confidence rarely experienced in other clinical areas. Gallop (1995) reports that patients feel most comfortable with interviewers who are: nonjudgmental, supportive, interested, and who listen carefully. Risen (1995) notes that your very willingness to discuss sexual matters offers patients an opportunity that society rarely provides. The ideal way of beginning the sexual history is to make a smooth transition from the social history. While patients are talking about relationships, dating, marriage, etc. it is usually easy to introduce questions about physical intimacy. Possible opening questions are:
- *What is the role of sexuality in your life right now?*
- *How would you describe your sexual relationships?*

Essentials of the Sexual History
Background
- *How was sexuality dealt with in your parents' home?*
- *When was your first partner-related sexual experience?*
- *What was it like for you?*

Activity
- *How important is sexuality in your life?*
- *When were you last sexually active?*
- *How often do you have sexual relations?*

Orientation
- *Are you attracted to men, women, or both?*
- *Are you sexually active with men, women, or both?*

Risk Factors
- *About how many sexual partners have you had?*
- *What kinds of activities do you engage in?*
- *What kinds of protection/ safe sex practices do you use?*
- *Have you been tested for HIV?*

Sexually Transmitted Diseases (STDs)
- *Have you ever had a sexually transmitted disease?* (you may have to list a couple to clarify the question)

Sexual Dysfunction
- *Do you have difficulties with any aspect of sexual activity?*

Risen (1995) lists a comprehensive scheme for taking a sexual history, which includes questions about:
- Comfort with gender identity
- Discovery of masturbation
- Experimentation as a child with other children
- Fantasies
- Paraphilic behavior

Structured questionnaires can be found in Lewis (1990) & Vollmer (1989).

Abuse

Physical and emotional abuse can be asked about with the following questions:
- *How did your parents react when you misbehaved?*
- *What kinds of punishment were used in your household?*
- *Were you punished out of proportion to what you did?*

Sexual abuse can be asked about as follows:
- *Were you ever touched by someone in a way you that you didn't like?*
- *Were you ever forced to do something sexually?*

Sexual abuse is common, but also commonly missed in interviews. In one survey, Briere (1989) found that 6% of women had **childhood sexual abuse (CSA)** recorded on their charts, while a rate of 70% was found for the same group when questions regarding CSA were posed directly. Gallop (1995) polled a group of nurses who had experienced CSA, and reported that the overall opinion was that not making inquiries about abuse reinforces the belief that it is a "dirty secret" that can't be shared, or that it is not important enough for a professional to ask about. It was also noted that some victims may not be ready to divulge CSA, and should not be pressured to discuss it if they so indicate. Figueroa (1997) investigated the presence of general psychopathology in victims of CSA. The parameters of abuse that were asked about were the following:

- Penetration
- Ongoing sexual abuse
- Sex with a parent
- Sex with a family member
- More than one perpetrator
- More than two perpetrators

These parameters were derived from the Family Experiences Interview (FEI) described in Silk (1995).

Legal History
Key Areas
- History of charges laid (for which crimes?)
- History of convictions (for which crimes?)
- Suspended sentences, probation or parole
- Offenses related to operating motor vehicles
- Upcoming court dates

Military History
Key Areas
- Branch of service
- Type of discharge
- Combat experience
- Injuries
- Disciplinary action taken
- Psychiatric referral

Obstetrical History

Key Areas
- Total number of pregnancies
- Number of term pregnancies
- Live births/ stillbirths
- Miscarriages/ abortions
- Adopted away children
- Postpartum psychiatric difficulties

Occupational/ Educational History

Key Areas
- School grades/ marks
- Highest level of education obtained, and why the person left at that time
- Number of jobs held, job description, responsibilities, and reasons for leaving
- Current position, description and responsibilities
- Recent changes in position at work; possibilities for advancement

References

J. Briere & L. Zaidi
Sexual Abuse Histories and Sequelae in Female Psychiatric Emergency Room Patients
American Journal of Psychiatry 146: p. 1602 — 1606, 1989

J.E. Ende, S. Rockwell & M. Glasgow
The Sexual History in General Medicine Practice
Archives of Internal Medicine 144: p. 558 — 561, 1984

E.F. Figueroa, K.R. Silk, A. Huth & N.E. Lohr
History of Childhood Sexual Abuse and General Psychopathology
Comprehensive Psychiatry 38: p. 23 — 30, 1997

R. Gallop, P. McKeever, B. Toner, W. Lancee & M. Lueck
Inquiring About Childhood Sexual Abuse as Part of the Nursing History: Opinions of Abused and Nonabused Nurses
Archives of Psychiatric Nursing 9: p. 146 — 151, 1995

The Psychiatric Interview — Explained

C.E. Lewis & H.E. Freeman
The Sexual History-taking and Counseling Practices of Primary Care Physicians
Western Journal of Medicine 147: p. 165 — 167, 1987

C.E. Lewis
Sexual Practices: Are Physicians Addressing the Issues?
Journal of General Internal Medicine 5(suppl): p. S78 — 81, 1990

W.C. Matthews & L.S. Linn
AIDS Prevention in Primary Care Clinics: Testing the Market
Journal of General Internal Medicine 4: p. 34 — 38, 1989

C.B. Risen
A Guide to Taking a Sexual History
The Psychiatric Clinics of North America 18: p. 39 — 53, 1995

K.R. Silk, S. Lee, E.M. Hill & N.E. Lohr
Borderline Personality Disorder Symptoms and Severity of Sexual Abuse
American Journal of Psychiatry 152: p. 1059 — 1064, 1995

S.A. Vollmer & K.B. Wells
The Preparedness of Freshman Medical Students For Taking Sexual Histories
Archives of Sexual Behavior 18: p. 167 — 177, 1989

11/ Review of Symptoms

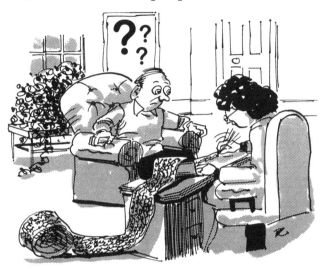

Introduction

The **Review of Symptoms (ROS)** can take place almost any-where in the interview. As stated, one advantage of taking it at just after the PersHx is that as you end up discussing the patient's current symptoms and stressors, so a smooth tran-sition can be made to the ROS.

Goals for the ROS

The ROS is a search for current symptoms that have not al-ready been identified in the HPI or other areas of the inter-view. This allows you to accomplish four goals:

- Further refine your hypothesis generation and testing
- Screening for the presence of other conditions that are not the focus of the patient's visit (e.g. phobias, etc.)

- Ask about symptoms of illnesses for which the patient is known to be at particular risk of developing because of historical, genetic, environmental or demographic factors elicited in the course of the interview
- Conduct a medical review of systems to further delineate general medical conditions, particularly those that can initiate or perpetuate a psychiatric illness

Points on Technique

A helpful way to introduce the ROS is to sum up the salient information you plan to use in your diagnostic formulation. As you finish reflecting them back to the patient, you can then go on to say something like:

Right now, I would like to shift our focus and ask about some other feelings and experiences that you may or may not have had. Sometimes there are conditions related to the problems you've described, and I would like to be as thorough as I possibly can be in understanding what is happening to you. I'll be asking about several different areas, so you can just say 'no' if what I'm asking about doesn't apply to you, and I'll go on to the next question.

An advantage of doing the ROS before the MSE is that it prepares patients for a wide range of questions, some of which you've acknowledged will not apply to the person directly. This helps take the awkwardness out of phrasing questions about parts of the MSE that are difficult to ask about (i.e. hallucinations and delusions).

Do I Ask About the Whole DSM-IV?

Thankfully, no. But it is at times difficult to know how far to cast your diagnostic net in the ROS. The following factors are a guide to which disorders should be included:

- Any condition in your list of differential diagnoses which you haven't fully inquired about

- New possibilities that have been discovered in the course of the history (e.g. posttraumatic stress disorder in some one whom you didn't initially know had seen combat)
- Conditions which are related to your principal diagnosis (e.g. for someone you think has panic disorder, ask about symptoms of the other anxiety disorders)
- Conditions which are among the most common epide-miologically

Screening Questions

Each DSM-IV diagnosis carries one or two essential symp-toms which define the disorder. These can be defined as "nec-essary but not sufficient" grounds for making the diagnosis. For example, everyone who suffers from a major depressive episode must experience a depressed mood or a loss of in-terest/ pleasure in activities. The presence of either of these symptoms alone cannot make the diagnosis, but one or both must be present along with other symptoms for the criteria to be met. The key to developing effective screening questions is to understand the essence of a disorder, and ask about these features in one or two questions.

Sample Questions

Psychotic Disorders
- *Do you ever have experiences that other people don't share, or that others consider unusual?*
- *Do you have strong ideas about things that other people either disagree with, or tell you cannot possibly be right?*
- *Do you feel your life is controlled by outside forces?*
- *Are you suspicious that others are out to harm you?*

Mania/ Hypomania
- *Have you had episodes where you were full of energy or ideas? Or that you felt high or extremely powerful?*
- *Did this episode last at least a week or longer?*

Phobias

- *Do you have strong fears about doing something embarrassing in front of other people? Do you avoid things like eating in public or speaking in front of others?*
- *Are there everyday things or situations you avoid because you have strong fears about them?*

Some clinicians pose questions which give more detail and several examples to give patients a clearer idea about what is being asked. Remember to avoid the use of jargon in the ROS — patients understand the term *fears* instead of *phobias* or *having visions* instead of *visual hallucinations*. The ROS can also be addressed by the use of structured interviews and self-report questionnaires. Some clinicians ask patients to complete symptom surveys before interviews. Self-report scales have the advantage of being economical to administer, can contain a wide range of questions, and can rate internal emotional states. Common self-report questionnaires are as follows:

- Hopkins Symptom Checklist 90R (SCL-90)
- General Health Questionnaire (GHQ)
- Zung Self-Rating Depression Scale (SDS)
- Beck Depression Inventory (BDI)
- State-Trait Anxiety Inventory (STAI)

Lishman (1998) provides an exceptional text for understanding the relationship between medical illnesses and psychiatric sequelae.

References

W.A. Lishman
Organic Psychiatry, Third Edition
Blackwell Science, Oxford, England, 1998

M. Zimmerman
A Five-Minute Psychiatric Screening Interview
The Journal of Family Practice 37: p. 479 — 482, 1993

12/ The Mental Status Exam

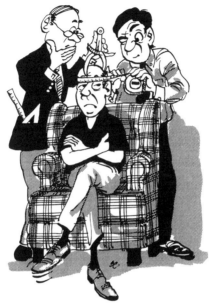

Introduction

The MSE is the component of an interview where cognitive functions are tested and inquiries are made about the symptoms of psychiatric conditions. It is a set of standardized observations and questions designed to evaluate sensorium, perception, thinking, feeling, and behavior. The MSE is an integral part of any clinical interview, not just one that takes place in a psychiatric context. An assessment of cognitive functioning must be made before information from patients can be considered accurate. The MSE records only observed behavior, cognitive abilities, and inner experiences expressed during the interview.

Points on Technique

The MSE begins as soon as the patient is in view. A moment of observation before the interview begins reveals important information such as: grooming, hygiene, behavior, gait, level of interest in and interaction with surroundings, etc. Invariably, there are items that will have to be specifically asked about, which can be done in one of the following ways:

- Take the opportunity when the chance arises in the interview, which is the most natural approach. This allows the MSE to be woven into the flow of the interview. For example, many patients will complain of poor memory and decreased attention span, presenting an ideal opportunity to test cognitive functioning.
- Take note of key points in the history that allow a smooth transition back to these items. For example, *You mentioned before that your vision was blurred. Did this ever cause you to see something unusual?*

The MSE can also be introduced as follows:
- *At this point, I'd like to ask you some questions that are separate from what we've been discussing so far, but will give me some important information about you*
- *Right now, I'd like to ask you some questions to give me an idea about some aspects of your mental functioning*
- *I'd like to switch now and ask you a set of questions that will help me evaluate your. . .(thinking, memory, etc.)*
- *There are some other areas that I need to formally test to get an idea about your. . .(concentration, attention, etc.)*

The MSE is explained in detail in another book from the 'Explained' series:
The Psychiatric Mental Status Exam — Explained
David J. Robinson, M.D.
ISBN 1-894328-20-5
© 2000, Rapid Psychler Press

How Do I Remember the Components of the Mental Status Exam?

A mnemonic can help. The following memory aid not only lists the main areas, but does so in the order that they are usually asked about and presented.

"ABC STAMP LICKER"

Appearance
Behavior
Cooperation

Speech
Thought — **form** and **content**
Affect — moment-to-moment variation in emotion
Mood — subjective emotional tone in the interview
Perception — in all sensory modalities

Level of consciousness
Insight & Judgment
Cognitive functioning & Sensorium
      Orientation
      Memory
      Attention & Concentration
      Reading & Writing
Knowledge base
Endings — suicidal and/ or homicidal ideation
Reliability of the information

The main sections, symptoms or findings from each of these areas will be presented in this section. A example of a write-up of the MSE appears in the Sample Case Report section in Appendix D, starting on page 120.

Appearance

- Actual & Apparent Age
- Attire
- Body Habitus
- Gender & Race
- Grooming & Hygiene
- Jewelry & Cosmetics
- Physical Abnormalities
- Other features, such as tattoos, body piercing, scars, unusual pattern of hair loss, etc.

Behavior

General Observations

- Agitation
- Hyperactivity
- Psychomotor Retardation

Observation of Specific Movements

- Akathisia
- Automatisms
- Catatonia
- Choreoathetoid Movements
- Compulsions
- Dystonias & Extrapyramidal Symptoms
- Negative Symptoms
- Tardive Dyskinesia
- Tics
- Tremors

Cooperation & Reliability

- Eye Contact
- Attitude/ Demeanor
- Attentiveness to the Interview
- Level of Consciousness
- Affect
- Secondary Gain

Speech

- Accent & Dialect
- Amount
- Aphasic Speech
- Modulation
- Pitch
- Rhythm/ Cadence
- Spontaneity

Thought Form/ Process

- Circumstantiality
- Clang Associations
- Echolalia
- Flight of Ideas
- Fragmentation
- Incoherence
- Jargon
- Loose Associations
- Neologisms
- Non sequiturs
- Perseveration
- Private use of words
- Punning
- Rambling
- Rate abnormalities
- Tangentiality
- Thought Blocking
- Thought Derailment
- Verbigeration
- Word Salad

Thought Content

- Delusions
  (erotomanic, grandiose, jealous, paranoid, passivity, control)
- Overvalued Ideas
- Obsessions
- Phobias
- Thoughts of Harm to Self or Others

Affect & Mood

Affect

- Type/ Quality
- Range/ Variability
- Degree/ Intensity
- Stability and Reactivity
- Appropriateness
- Congruence
    - to Mood
    - to Appearance
    - to Behavior

Mood

- Quality/ Type
- Reactivity
- Intensity
- Stability/ Duration

Perception

- Hallucinations
- Illusions
- Disturbances of Self and Environment
- Disturbances of Quality or Size
- Disturbances in the Intensity of Perception
- Disturbances of Experience

Insight & Judgment

Cognitive Functioning

- Orientation
- Attention & Concentration
- Memory
    - (Immediate, Recent, Remote)
- Intelligence Estimation
- Knowledge Base/ Fund of Information
- Capacity to Read and Write
- Abstraction/ Concrete Thinking
- Visuospatial Ability

A/ *Thoughts of Harm to Self & Others*

Introduction

Asking about thoughts of self harm or violent intentions is often fraught with apprehension because of the delicacy required in phrasing questions and the consequences of either being present. Yet the findings in the history or MSE pale in significance if the patient or someone else is going to come to harm.

In recognition that the majority of those who commit suicide suffer from a mental disorder, suicidal ideation is almost universally grounds for involuntary committal.

Conversely, most violent crime is not perpetrated by those who are psychiatrically ill. The provision of civil commitment on the grounds of harm to another is made to detain those who have a "defect in reasoning." Such a defect is frequently due to the presence of a formal thought disorder, such as perceptual aberrations (e.g. hallucinations) or (most often) due to paranoid delusions. Patients who have plans to harm someone as a result of their mental illness require protection, as do their intended victims.

Mental health professionals are continually faced having to predict the likelihood of future violence. Patients' intentions to harm themselves or someone else impacts at the start of a treatment plan. (Do I admit this person to hospital? Should he or she be involuntarily committed?)

The following mnemonic covers key elements in assessing suicidal risk:

"SADDLE SORE WOMAN"

Social isolation (Section I)
Age (II)
Disturbed interpersonal relationships (DIRs) (III)
Drug use/ abuse (IV)
Lethality of method (V)
Ethanol use (VI)

Sex (VII)
Occupation (VIII)
Repeated attempts (IX)
Event — acute precipitant (X)

Will — created or altered (XI)
Organic condition — chronic medical illness (XII)
Mental illness (XIII)
Antidepressant use (XIV)
Note written (XV)

(I) Social Isolation, in general, refers to a sense of *unconnectedness* with others. This can be in terms of marital status, occupation or even patients' view of themselves. Suicide rates are higher for people who live alone. Many people who live alone prefer the solitude and freedom from distraction that this provides. Before listing this as a risk factor, it is important to know if it is a patient's choice to live alone, and how great a departure this is from desired living arrangements.

(II) Age is a factor because certain age groups are statistically correlated with a higher risk of completed suicides. As a general rule, the prevalence of suicide increases with age. This trend clearly develops in men starting at about age 45, and climbs continually, with a peak at age 75. Women have a later onset, starting around age 55 and exhibit a less dramatic rise with age. The elderly have a suicide rate triple that of younger people, and commit one-quarter of all suicides while encompassing only one-tenth of the population.

There is an important exception to this trend. The suicide rate among males aged 15-24 years is disproportionately high (especially among whites). In this age group, suicide is consistently reported to be either the second or third most common cause of death (with accidents and homicide being the other causes). While no clear reason has been established, it has been suggested that the prevalence of alcohol and drug abuse is a significant factor. Peer pressure and exposure to media depictions of suicide are also thought to be relevant factors.

(III) Disturbed Interpersonal Relationships (DIRs). Disruptions in meaningful relationships provide perhaps the best answer as to *why* people take their lives. **DIRs** are one of the most common, if not *the* major cause of visits to emergency rooms for emotional reasons. DIRs in particular refer to:
- The threat of rejection or abandonment
- Loss of approval, acceptance, affection or attachment

(IV) Drug use/ abuse is strongly correlated with completed suicide when the drugs used (or available) are highly lethal when taken in overdose. Those with the greatest potential to cause death are:
- Amphetamines
- Cocaine
- Barbiturates
- Opioids

In some cases, the term *drugs* refers to illicit substances or street drugs, and *medication* to those obtained by prescription. It is important to ask about both prescription and non-prescription drug use, though all but cocaine from the above list can be obtained by a physician's order.

The greatest risk appears to be through combining drugs of abuse (including alcohol). A common situation involves using certain drugs to modulate or prolong highs, reduce distractions, and to avoid the dysphoria of "crashes."

The prevalence of drug use among adolescents and young adults is thought to be a major contributor to the increased rates of suicide seen in this age group. The presence of certain factors involving the use of substances increases the risk:

- Early age of onset
- Chronic use
- Past overdoses
- Male gender
- Family history of substance abuse

(V) Lethality of the method is another factor that bears on the risk of suicide. In general, the more lethal the means, the more likely it will be carried out. Males tend to use violent methods, such as firearms, knives, jumping and hanging. Females are more likely to take overdoses, drown, or asphyxiate themselves. The availability of firearms has been shown to have an impact on the suicide rate.

(VI) Ethanol use can lead to problems during intoxication or withdrawal states. Alcohol deserves special mention because it is the substance most often associated with acts of violence. Ethanol causes disinhibition and removes the self-restraint that would otherwise be present. The combination of impaired judgment with a greater propensity to take action has dire consequences. It is common in emergency rooms to have intoxicated patients who are combative or self-destructive, yet become entirely different when sober.

(VII) Sex (gender) is unevenly distributed for attempts and completed suicides. In all age ranges, males commit suicide more frequently than females. The ratio varies from a factor of 2:1 to almost 10:1 depending on the age group and race. Two factors help explain the gender discrepancy. As outlined in the 'L' (lethality) section, males use more lethal methods. The time course of an overdose, asphyxiation or drowning allows an intervention to be made. Only seconds to minutes are available for someone to intervene when more lethal means are used. Secondly, males have a higher prevalence of chemical dependency. In North America, the ratio of males to females with alcohol problems is at least 4:1. In other areas of the world it is considerably higher.

(VIII) Occupation. Employment is a protective factor. Higher socio-economic status is associated with higher risk (though a recent change in status is also a risk factor). A possible explanation is that a higher level of occupation generally requires increased responsibility. Professionals, and in particular, physicians are generally above national averages. Recent studies have indicated that female physicians have rates triple the national average for women over age 25.

(IX) Repeated attempts at self-harm increase the risk of a completed suicide. A distinction needs to be made between past serious, unsuccessful attempts and chronic thoughts of suicide or gestures of self-harm. The latter occurrence is called **parasuicide** and refers to chronic self-mutilation, persistent thoughts or threats of suicide, or non-lethal attempts.

- Those that demographically are at higher risk for completed suicide are older males who are socially isolated, use a method of high lethality, and who have either a mood disorder or a chemical dependency.
- Attempters tend to be younger women who have some social connections, use methods that are unlikely to be fatal (and likely to be discovered), and have a personality disorder or adjustment disorder.

Women attempt suicide more frequently than men, though men complete more suicides. Most attempts occur in younger age groups, which is the opposite to the picture for completed suicides. Attempts are made impulsively, whereas completed suicides are more often planned and take place in settings with a low chance of discovery or rescue. Among attempters, a personality disorder has been reported to be the most common diagnosis, with borderline and antisocial personality disorder most prominently featured. With borderline personalities in particular, parasuicidal behavior can become a way of life as a means to manipulate others.

(X) Events of an acute nature increase the risk of suicide. The presence of *loss* is central to precipitants that lead to suicidal behavior. This can be perceived or actual loss of love, esteem, wealth, health, fame, etc. The most common event leading to the wish to die is a disturbance in an interpersonal relationship (DIR).

Searching for the "final straw" is a valuable endeavor when assessing suicidal patients. It is important to understand *why* the patient made an attempt or is considering suicide *at this point in time*. There is almost always an explanation for why patients do not want to go on living. Most people at least transiently consider suicide at some point. Traumatic events like the death of a spouse, child or parent frequently cause surviving parties to consider whether their own lives are worthwhile. Some statistics on suicide are as follows:
- 20% of adults have persistent thoughts of suicide over a 2 week period
- 10% of adults have made a plan as to how they would commit suicide
- 3% of adults have made an attempt at suicide

In situations where a precipitant is not obvious, consideration of three other factors may help:
1. In some cases, people react to a symbolic loss rather than an actual one. Exploring the meaning of apparently minor losses can help identify a precipitant.
2. People may not be consciously aware of what influences them. For example, watching a movie or hearing a song can bring about associations that evoke painful memories.
3. Anniversary reactions occur on the dates of major losses. Some patients may be completely unaware of why they are

suicidal at a certain point in time. An exploration of dates significant to that person may reveal this as the cause.

(XI) Wills and **Notes** indicate that planning is involved, which increases the risk of a completed suicide. Patients who wish to "tidy up their affairs" may have wills created or altered. Many patients make reference to their will, or changes in it, prior to a suicide attempt.

(XII) Organic conditions (general medical conditions) can be risk factors due to their seriousness or chronicity. This is also one of the reasons why suicide is more frequent in the elderly. A list of conditions associated with increased risk is as follows:

Central Nervous System
- Dementia (of any type)
- Degenerative Conditions
- Epilepsy
- Head injuries
- Strokes

Cancer
- particularly those that grow quickly or are advanced at the time of discovery

Musculoskeletal
- Amputations

Cardiovascular
- Unstable angina

Gastrointestinal
- Peptic ulcer
- Inflammatory bowel disease
- Cirrhosis
- Porphyria

Renal
- Dialysis dependence

Endocrine
- Cushing's Disease

HIV Seropositivity or **AIDS**

(XIII) Mental Illness is the strongest risk factor associated with suicide. Over 90% of those who take their own lives have a diagnosable mental condition at the time of death. The presence of a mental illness is estimated to increase the risk of committing suicide tenfold. The majority of patients who commit suicide have seen a physician within six months of their death, and frequently within one month. Other studies have found that a high percentage of patients who took their lives had been given a prescription for psychotropic medication. Among psychiatric disorders, mood disorders and alcohol abuse are the conditions that have the highest association with suicide (respectively). Other conditions/ factors are:

Mood Disorders
* Depression with psychotic features
* Bipolar mixed states (the co-existence of manic and depressive symptoms; of particular concern is that the high energy state of mania can cause patients to act on the suicidal thoughts brought about by depression)

Schizophrenia
* Young males appear to be at particular risk, especially early in the course of the illness
* Patients with high premorbid achievement and personal expectations pose a high risk for completed suicide
* Recovery from a psychotic episode, especially during a postpsychotic depression
* Patients with an awareness of the overall prognosis
* Patients with the additional risk factors of social isolation and substance abuse

Personality Disorders (PDs)
* Antisocial and Borderline PDs

(IV) Antidepressants typically bring about recovery in a certain sequence:
With Tricyclic Antidepressants (TCAs):
* Insomnia and appetite may improve within 7 days

With selective serotonin reuptake inhibitors (SSRIs):
• Energy and interest may improve within 7 days

The overall recovery tends to follow a pattern of vegetative symptoms recovering first, then cognitive functions, and lastly, mood symptoms and suicidal thoughts. The recovery sequence can place patients in the situation where they have an increase in energy level concurrent with thoughts of self-harm.

What Other Aspects of Suicidal Risk Need to be Assessed?

Another important factor is **family history**. There are studies that demonstrate a genetic inheritance independent of other major risk factors (mood disorders, schizophrenia and alcoholism). Twin studies show a higher concordance rate for suicide in monozygotic twins than dizygotic twins. Additionally, adoption studies have found increased rates of completed suicide among the biological relatives of adopted away off-spring, furthering the speculation of a genetic contribution. Patients who, particularly under the age of ten, lost a parent to suicide are at an increased risk themselves through the process of **identification** with the deceased. A parent's suicide seems to break the "taboo" in families, and in a sense, transmit that suicide is acceptable when things get tough. This is one of the ways that the tragedy of suicide perpetuates itself. Patients who have lost parents to suicide may not only suffer from **anniversary reactions**, but also be involved unconsciously in a self-destructive process at the same age as the parent who died.

How Do I Ask About Violent Intentions?

Patients may not be open and honest about their intentions in this regard. For this reason, clinicians need to keep an index of suspicion about the possibility of violence and use all available sources of information. Current stressors of a financial or interpersonal nature are common precipitants for taking action against others. The best predictor of violent behavior is a history of such behavior. Sample questions that can be asked are as follows:

- *Have you had thoughts about wanting to get revenge on someone? Did you ever develop a plan?*
- *Are you currently having any ideas about wanting to hurt someone? Do you have a particular person in mind?*
- *What would you do if you met a person you didn't like?*
- *Do you have access to guns, knives or other weapons?*

Conditions Most Frequently Associated With Violence
"MADS & BADS"

Mania — at risk due to impulsivity, grandiosity, high energy level, and possible psychotic symptoms

Alcohol — due to intoxication (disinhibition) or withdrawal states (altered perception and irritability)

Dementia — poor judgment and disinhibition

Schizophrenia — most common with the paranoid subtype; command hallucinations or delusions also elevate the risk

Borderline Personality Disorder— intense anger and unstable emotions can be part of a rage reaction when abandonment occurs or is perceived to take place

Antisocial Personality Disorder — disregard for the safety of others; sadistic enjoyment of the suffering of others

Delirium — hallucinations and delusions can cause violent reactions (usually in a disorganized fashion)

Substance Abuse — intoxication, particularly with hallucinogens and PCP (phencyclidine)

B/ *Before the Interview*

Preparing the Room

The interview room must provide the necessities for your evaluation, facilitate your ability to concentrate, and be free from distractions. If at all possible, speak with patients in a private room. Interviews conducted in hallways (e.g. due to overcrowded rooms in emergency departments) are almost always unsatisfactory for reasons of confidentiality. You cannot ask the questions crucial to an assessment, and patients are certainly going to be guarded about sharing information when others can overhear the interview.

Arranging your seat at approximately a 45-degree angle to the patient's seat helps avoid continuous face-to-face contact, which many people find inhibiting or even threatening. Chairs should be available for everyone in the room. Patients may start speaking to anyone sitting in front of them, so observers are best seated in the periphery to minimize possible distraction. Sitting in front of a clock will help you keep track of time. If this is not possible, you can either position your watch so it faces up, or purchase a watch or timer that can attach to your clipboard. Making obvious glances at your wristwatch is distracting to patients.

Preparing Yourself

Interviewing is hard work. Balancing diagnostic possibilities with process techniques while investigating cues as you elicit emotional responses is taxing! Take a few minutes to prepare yourself so you will be ready:

- When nature calls, answer — you can't concentrate with persistent, intrusive thoughts of the washroom dominating your consciousness
- Have a snack and a beverage before speaking with patients

- Sign over your pager before the interview
- Assemble your forms, pages, clipboard, pens, etc. before entering the room
- Make a phone call or two to clear up pressing matters so you won't be preoccupied during the interview

Safety Concerns

The issue of whether mentally ill patients are more likely to be violent than those in the general population has been a cause for debate in the literature. Some research has been conducted to combat the stigma that all psychiatric patients have a high propensity for violent acts. Methodological flaws and differences in definition make a global conclusion difficult to reach (e.g. comparing violent acts on inpatient wards vs. those occurring in the community). However, there is no debate about the fact that patients with mental illnesses *can* be violent, and that all clinicians need to develop a "situational awareness" about their risk of being harmed.

In emergency situations, it is advisable that at least two staff members sit in on the interview. If this is not possible, inform others that you are going to conduct an interview and ask them to check in on you. Hospital security or police officers can also be present during your assessment. You cannot conduct a good interview if you are distracted by safety concerns.

Even in cases where the sounds of an assault will be heard, other hospital staff may be reluctant to intrude, or may take a few minutes to assemble.

Be constantly attuned to the safety aspects of your interview.

C/ Winding Down the Interview

Just as an interview needs a "warm up," a moment spent winding down at the end of the assessment is quite beneficial. At the end of the interview, you will have asked a lot of questions and found out a considerable amount about your patient. Some of this information is used in formulating a treatment plan, and some of it is useful for building a therapeutic alliance with either yourself or the next person involved in the patient's care. Abrupt endings to interviews are awkward and potentially detrimental to the rapport you've developed. Ending interviews is a matter of personal preference. Suggestions for particular situations are as follows:

When You Are Continuing to Treat the Patient
- Acknowledge that the interview has been thorough and potentially draining for the patient, and then ask how he or she feels at the moment
- Ask if there is anything you've omitted that the patient thinks you should know, or that requires clarification
- Discuss the treatment plan (e.g. investigations, next appointment, etc.)

When Someone Else is Going to Treat the Patient
- Employ the first and second steps from above
- Discuss the next step in the treatment plan, who will be taking over the patient's care, and when this will take place

Examination Situations
- Thank the patient for spending the time to help you with the exam
- Ask the patient what his or her plans are, and offer your "best wishes" or "good luck" for the future

D/ Sample Case Report

I.D.   Mr. Dexter Smyth is a 33-year-old, white male. He is single (never married), has no children, and follows the Catholic faith. He is unemployed and is currently homeless.

RFR: Mr. Smyth was accosting patrons outside a shopping center and was brought to the emergency department by police.

HPI: Mr. Smyth was last known to be functioning at his usual level about three weeks ago. At that time, the opportunity to renew the lease on his apartment was denied by his landlord (Mr. Crump). Mr. Crump was apparently upset at Mr. Smyth's poor payment history, intermittent playing of country music, and possible drug use.

In the three weeks since leaving his apartment, Mr. Smyth has been alternating nights at hostels and on park benches. He thinks that his landlord found some important evidence in his apartment regarding a government conspiracy, and now there are secret agents monitoring his activities. Mr. Smyth feels he must keep moving to try and elude them because he can hear occasional radio transmissions that indicate he is being pursued. He avoids stores because he thinks he'll be recorded on their security systems. He was desperate for cigarettes, and wanted to quickly get some from mall patrons so he could leave the area prior to the police arriving.

Evaluation of psychotic symptoms reveals that Mr. Smyth is having intermittent auditory hallucinations that sound like a group of people talking over a radio. He doesn't recognize the voices, and they don't tell him to do anything in particular. He wasn't around any radios when he heard them. These experiences occur unpredictably, and he heard this radio chatter at various times during the interview.

He is completely convinced that he was being pursued, and would be kept in detention and interrogated if caught. Mr. Smyth has been keeping track of winning lottery numbers and has developed a formula to predict them. He thinks the government was told about his frequent "research trips" to local stores to record winning numbers and his borrowing books on statistics from public libraries. He did not endorse any concerns about his health (somatic delusions) or about anyone being envious of his formula (delusions of jealousy). He did not have any grandiose plans for the money, wasn't interested in getting anyone's attention with it, and was unsure how he'd spend it. He did not speak or behave in an obviously odd manner.

He does admit to feeling depressed, but only since yesterday when his cigarettes ran out. He does, at other times, feel down for as long as a week at a time. He does not feel speeded up, energized, or as if he has any special powers. He is irritable, somewhat distractible, and said he'd slept very little lately.

PPH: Mr. Smyth was first hospitalized at age 19 shortly after his freshman year in college, where he was studying mathematics. He found it very stressful to be away from his family. He was living in residence at the time, and was occasionally teased because he felt awkward around others and didn't socialize well. About six weeks before his finals, he spent all his time in isolation studying. He felt he was not going to be ready for exams and started taking amphetamines to aid his preparation. After his last exam, he became extremely agitated, suspicious of others, and hostile. He was hospitalized involuntarily shortly afterwards. This admission lasted one month, and upon release he agreed to take antipsychotic medication.

He has had two other admissions, eight and four years ago, respectively. He typically gets admitted for disturbing others. He's felt persecuted for years and at times sees the people who are after him. He has never acknowledged having an illness, and does not take medication on a regular basis.

MedHx: Mr. Smyth has not had a physical check-up since his last admission four years ago. He does not have a family doctor, and cannot recall if he has any physical illnesses. He had one episode of loss of consciousness in a car accident in his mid-teens. He denies any allergies and does not have a medic-alert bracelet. He does not take prescription medication. He admits to taking over-the-counter analgesics (acetaminophen) and other pills which help him sleep (dimenhydrinate). He takes up to ten per night of the latter, and has been doing so since he left his apartment (his most recent use of this medication was last night). He subsists on a diet of fast food, snack food, and coffee. He is underweight and does not exercise.

SubHx: Mr. Smyth admits to taking street drugs on an intermittent basis. His substance use can be heavy when drugs are available, but he does not take anything on a continual basis. He admits to taking marijuana, amphetamines, magic mushrooms, PCP, and LSD. His last use of any illicit substance was 2 days ago and involved about 10 hits of LSD. He either smokes or swallows drugs, and denies ever using injections. He does not experience withdrawal symptoms when he doesn't "use" for an extended period. He's smoked heavily since his first admission. He uses minimal amounts of caffeine and alcohol.

FamHx: Mr. Smyth is an only child. His parents are both alive and live in a city one hour away. Mr. Smyth's father works as an IRS auditor, has some difficulties with arthritis, but is otherwise healthy and has never seen a psychiatrist. Mr. Smyth's mother is physically well, but she suffered a "breakdown" shortly after his birth and did not return to work as a computer programmer. She sees a psychiatrist, but the details of her treatment are unknown. Mr. Smyth's maternal aunt and her son have both been diagnosed with schizophrenia, but again the details about these two people are lacking.

PersHx: Mr. Smyth was born in New York. He was a term delivery, born in late January in a hospital. There was some concern about his health at birth (possible anoxia). He recalls being told that forceps were required, and that he had a low APGAR. He met his developmental milestones appropriately, and had no childhood or adolescent difficulties that required psychiatric intervention. He described his childhood as being fairly isolative. Though his mother was at home, she had a limited tolerance for his interests and energy, and persuaded him to find quiet activities such as reading. His father was a good provider, but had little interest in doing anything once he got home. His father's interests were largely quiet solitary pursuits, such as crossword puzzles and stamp collecting. Owing to his father's occupation, Mr. Smyth felt that he was ostracized by neighbors, and had few friends. He did not participate in team sports.

In high school, he obtained above-average marks. His particular interests were mathematics, philosophy, chess, and astronomy. He went with a neighbor's daughter to his high school graduation, but did not date otherwise. He entered college with the hope of becoming an actuary. He reports no episodes of sexual or physical abuse. He was punished primarily by having to "justify" his actions, and recalls feeling guilty most of his life. He describes himself as heterosexual, and has had a couple of brief relationships with female patients he's met while in hospital. He did not serve in the military. Other than pending charges for loitering, he was charged with assault for an altercation before his admission four years ago. He failed his first year final exams and has not returned to college. He worked at a series of entry-level jobs, but stayed for one to two months in all cases. He missed shifts and had difficulty dealing with the public.

ROS: Symptoms were asked about the following disorders:

- depression
- mania
- schizophrenia
- substance abuse/ dependence
- antisocial personality disorder
- delusional disorder

MSE

- Appearance: tattered jeans, soiled sneakers, and a sweater which seemed too heavy for the warm weather; unshaven with unwashed hair; tobacco stains on hands
- Behavior: restless during the interview, stood up twice to look in the ashtray, but was able to be directed back to his seat; fidgeted constantly with his lighter and appeared distracted
- Cooperation: moderately interested in the interview; information limited but considered reliable; eye contact was continuous
- Speech: spontaneous and fluent, spoke in a low voice and had occasional difficulty naming people, places, and events
- Thought Content: answered questions with little elaboration; spontaneously spoke about the injustices he'd suffered by "the system" and specified how today's events were part of a scheme to persecute him; this belief was strongly held throughout the interview and unwavering in intensity
- Thought Process: his thoughts were logically connected with a restricted flow of ideas; one episode of thought derailment
- Affect & Mood: his emotional expression ranged from mildly sullen to moderately irritable; he became hostile when told he would have to remain in the hospital; he described his mood as "p***ed off" and reported it as a one out of ten
- Perception: experienced clearly formed auditory hallucinations in the interview which he says reported his location; in response

to this he wanted to be released immediately; he did not report perceptual disturbances in other sensory modalities

- Suicide/ Homicide: no thoughts or plans for self-harm, he wishes to assault one of the officers who brought him to hospital
- Insight & Judgment: impaired, denies he was bothering anyone or has any need for hospitalization or treatment
- Cognition
  · alert and fully conscious throughout the interview
  · oriented to person, day, date, month, year, season, and place
  · able to register three objects on the second attempt and recall two of them four minutes later (despite prompting, he couldn't recall the third); remote memory was impaired for historical details obtained from hospital record (dates and events)
  · digit span — five forward, four backward; attempted two serial seven subtractions both were incorrect (97, 87), then stopped this task
  · declined to answer questions testing general knowledge, abstraction ability, or proverb interpretation

Diagnostic Formulation

Mr. Dexter Smyth is a 33-year-old, single, homeless, white male. He has a history of serious mental illness starting at age 19, when he had to be hospitalized on an involuntary basis for agitation and hostility. He has been hospitalized twice since then, and has been charged with assault prior to one hospitalization. He currently presents with a three-week history of auditory hallucinations, persecutory delusions, and increasing disorganization. He has an extensive and varied substance use history, and admits to taking 10 hits of LSD two days ago, and 10 dimenhydrinate tablets nightly for three weeks. He indicates that the hallucinations and delusions persist even when he is not using any street drugs. He does exhibit some depressive symptoms and some of a manic-like quality. There were indications that he has cognitive impairment, which could affect the accuracy of his history.

Preferred Diagnosis: • Schizophrenia, Paranoid Type
                        • Substance Abuse (hallucinogens and anticholinergic medications

Differential Diagnosis: • Substance-Induced Psychotic Disorder (hallucinogens and anticholinergic agents)

- Schizoaffective Disorder, Depressive Type
- Depressive Episode with Mood-Incongruent Psychotic Features
- Bipolar Mood Disorder, Most Recent Episode Mixed, with Psychotic Features

Etiologic Formulation

	Predisposing	Precipitating	Perpetuating
Biological	· genetic loading · birth anoxia? · season of birth	· substance use · poor health and nutrition	· substance use · noncompliance with medication
Psychological	· low self esteem · lack of parental involvement · punitive superego	· stressful exam period · fear of failing in exams	· lack of insight into condition · hostility towards others
Social	· difficulties making friends · ostracized by neighborhood	· isolation from family · teasing from other students	· lack of friends or intimate rel'n · lacks vocational skills

Biopsychosocial Management Plan

1. Admit to hospital on an involuntary basis

Investigations	Biological	Complete physical exam, bloodwork (CBC, thyroid tests, Vitamin B_{12}, folate), urine test for substances of abuse
	Social	Collateral history, ADL and IADL assessment
	Psychological	Further investigation of cognitive deficits
Short Term Treatment	Biological	Antipsychotic medication
	Social	Assistance in finding housing (preferably in a group home); ascertain parental interest
	Psychological	Possible Behavior Therapy; inpatient Group Therapy; Recreation Therapy
Longer-Term Treatment	Biological	Adjust dose/ switch medication; consider a depot antipsychotic
	Social	Education about drug use and his illness
	Psychological	Case manager; ongoing support group

Index

The Author

Dave Robinson is a psychiatrist practicing in London, Ontario, Canada. His particular interests are consultation-liaison psychiatry, undergraduate and postgraduate education. He is a graduate of the University of Toronto Medical School and is a Lecturer in the Department of Psychiatry at the University of Western Ontario in London, Canada.

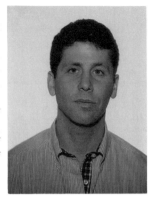

The Artist

Brian Chapman is a resident of Oakville, Ontario, Canada. He was born in Sussex, England and moved to Canada in 1957. Brian was formerly a Creative Director at Mediacom. He continues to freelance and is versatile in a wide range of media. He is a master of the caricature, and his talents are constantly in demand.

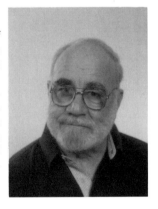

Rapid Psychler Press

Rapid Psychler Press was founded in 1994 with the aim of producing textbooks and resource materials that further the use of humor in mental health education. In addition to textbooks, Rapid Psychler Press specializes in producing slides and overheads for presentations.